The Secret Raven

Marie-Louise von Franz, Honorary Patron

**Studies in Jungian Psychology
by Jungian Analysts**

Daryl Sharp, General Editor

# The Secret Raven

## CONFLICT AND TRANSFORMATION
### in the life of
### FRANZ KAFKA

DARYL SHARP

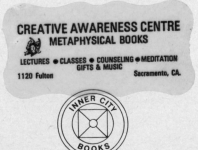

INNER CITY
BOOKS

For Tony, Dick, and Pit

Canadian Cataloguing in Publication Data

Sharp, Daryl, 1936–
    The secret raven

(Studies in Jungian psychology)
Includes index.
ISBN 0-919123-00-7

1.  Kafka, Franz, 1883–1924—Biography—Character.
2.  Authors, Austrian—20th century—Biography.
I.  Title.  II.  Series.

PT2621.A26Z87        833'.912      C80-090054-5

INNER CITY BOOKS
Box 1271, Station Q, Toronto, Canada M4T 2P4

Honorary Patron: Marie-Louise von Franz

Cover: Detail of a drawing in *Letters to Milena* (see text page 41).

Set in Theme by Blain Berdan, Toronto.
Printed and bound in Canada by Webcom Limited

# CONTENTS

Ich schreibe das ganz bestimmt aus Verzweiflung über meinen Körper und über die Zukunft mit diesem Körper

Wenn sich die Verzweiflung so bestimmt gibt so an ihren Gegenstand gebunden ist, so zurückgehalten wie von einem Soldaten, der den Rückzug deckt und sich dafür zerreissen lässt, dann ist es nicht die richtige Verzweiflung. Die richtige Verzweiflung hat ihr Ziel gleich und immer überholt. (Bei diesem Beistrich zeigte es sich, dass nur der erste Satz richtig war)

A Manuscript Page from Kafka's *Diaries* (May, 1910)

> I don't believe people exist whose inner plight
> resembles mine; still, it is possible for me to
> imagine such people — but that the secret raven
> forever flaps about their heads as it does about
> mine, even to imagine that is impossible.
>
> — *Diaries,* October 17, 1921

## Introduction

Franz Kafka was born in Prague in 1883, the son of a rich Czech merchant. He died of tuberculosis in 1924, not yet 41 years old.

Although a Czech, all Kafka's writings were in German. He wrote three novels — *America, The Trial,* and *The Castle* — all more or less unfinished, and a lot of short stories and fragmentary narratives. Very little of his work, including his diaries (covering the years 1910-1923), was published during his lifetime. Everything he wrote, and particularly his diaries, is an account of his struggles to cope with not only the ultimate mysteries, but even the basic realities of everyday life.

It is said that Thomas Mann once lent a book by Kafka to Albert Einstein, who returned it with the comment: "I couldn't read it, the human mind isn't complicated enough."[1] Angel Flores, editor of *The Kafka Problem,* a collection of critical essays, mentions this anecdote and goes on to say:

> If Einstein finds Kafka beyond his understanding, he is the
> only man who has ever admitted it. Nearly everyone who reads
> Kafka, not to mention many who don't, seems to have not the
> slightest doubt that he understands him perfectly, and more-
> over that he is the only one who does.[2]

It is abundantly clear that there is no consensus about either Kafka the man or Kafka the artist. He has been compared or contrasted with Charles Dickens, Gogol, Nietzsche, Dostoyevski, Kierkegaard, Karl Barth, Herman Melville, and Ernest Hemingway, among others. He has been called neurotic, psychotic, abnormal, pathological, perverse, and schizophrenic on the one hand, and on the other he has been hailed as a major religious writer of the twentieth century. And there are all shades of opinion in between.

C.G. Jung has suggested that the struggle to express an inner vision of a reality greater than the individual self, a reality that transcends the mundane, is what lies at the root of the genuine artistic impulse.[3] I believe that it is pertaining to this struggle — essentially religious — that Kafka has his primary significance as a writer. But as an individual, Kafka's fate was altogether more banal, in that most of his life was lived "provisionally," due to a conflict between the demands of his inner world and his aspirations in outer reality.

In this respect Kafka was a man of his and our time; his neurosis, the "provisional life," as an aspect of the *puer aeternus* problem, was and is the neurosis of the modern age. It is not by any means confined to artists. The difference is that the artist may exploit it, may even make a living through it, while the ordinary man, and the artist whose creative work does not support him — like Kafka — will make a living only in spite of it.

The expression *puer aeternus* (literally, "eternal child") derives originally from Greek mythology, where it designates a child-god who is forever young (e.g., Iacchus, Dionysus, Eros). My use of it in this study is substantially based on the concept as it is developed by Marie-Louise von Franz, for many years Jung's co-worker and herself an analyst, in her book, *The Problem of the Puer Aeternus.* "In general," she writes,

> the man who is identified with the archetype of the *puer aeternus* remains too long in adolescent psychology; that is, all those characteristics that are normal in a youth of seventeen or eighteen are continued into later life, coupled in most cases with too great a dependence on the mother.[4]

The term *puer* must be understood as descriptive rather than pejorative. It is necessary to stress this due to the widespread misconception, even among Jungians, that it is a damning appellation. In fact, the expression *puer* is used psychologically to personify certain typical attitudes and behaviour patterns that are present in everyone. The task, in what Jung has called the individuation process, is to consciously relate to these attitudes (among others), rather than identifying with them. Identification is not something one does deliberately, it simply exists as a given state of affairs; it appears as one-sidedness, and one-sidedness is perhaps the most common symptom of neurosis.

What all this has to do with Kafka will become clear in the course of this book. My aim has not been to explain or interpret Kafka's creative work. Rather I have tried to illuminate some of the psychological factors involved in his conflicts, paying special attention to the compensatory significance of some of his dreams.

Nor is it any part of my intention, by delving into Kafka's personal psychology, to diminish his stature as an artist. Kafka's art rises above the personal, and speaks, in Jung's words, "from the mind and heart of the artist to the mind and heart of mankind."[5]

A Manuscript Page from Kafka's *Diaries* (May, 1910)

# PART ONE:
# BIOGRAPHICAL

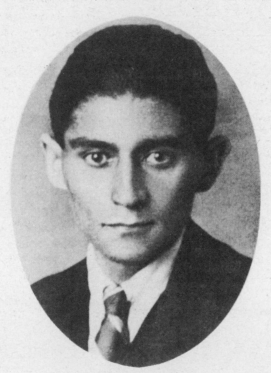

FRANZ KAFKA
1883 — 1924

# 1  WORK

Kafka received his Doctorate in law from Prague University in 1906, at the age of 23. He had chosen to study law, according to his friend and biographer Max Brod, because it involved "the least fixed goal, or the largest choice of goals,"[6] and was most likely to be of practical use in the business of earning a living. It was never his intention to practice as a lawyer, nor did he ever do so. His one ambition was to write.

After a false start in a hectic commercial office, he joined the staff of a semi-government agency, the Workers Accident Insurance Institute for the Kingdom of Bohemia. This promised to be exactly what he was looking for: the hours were not long, the work itself neither difficult nor demanding. His duties were primarily to look into the causes of accidents and the amount of risk involved in the various trades. It had only one drawback: it was, after all, a regular job.

Although Kafka held the same position for more than twelve years, the effort it cost him is evident from any number of anguished diary entries, an avalanche of despair and self-pity at his continually frustrated attempts to find enough time free to write.

In December, 1910, he notes:

> That I, so long as I am not freed of my office, am simply lost, that is clearer to me than anything else, it is just a matter, as long as it is possible, of holding my head so high that I do not drown. (D1 35)*

---

*Page references to Kafka's diaries are from *The Diaries of Franz Kafka*, 1910-1913 (D1) and 1914-1923 (D2).

More often than not, he arrived home mentally and physically exhausted, miserable with frustration. "I am too tired," runs a typical diary entry:

> I must try to rest and sleep, otherwise I am lost in every respect.
> What an effort to keep alive! Erecting a monument does not re-
> quire the expenditure of so much strength. (D2 23)

He tried sleeping when he had an afternoon off and writing at night, but that meant drawing on his last reserves of strength to get through the next day. "I won't give up the diary again," he writes at one point, "I must hold on here, it is the only place I can." (D1 33)

Recording a conversation in 1911 with Dr. Rudolph Steiner, the anthroposophist, Kafka explained the apparent hopelessness of his situation. His job and his writing, he said, were "two never-to-be-reconciled endeavours":

> The smallest good fortune in one becomes a great misfortune
> in the other. If I have written something good one evening, I am
> afire the next day in the office and can bring nothing to com-
> pletion. This back and forth continually becomes worse. Out-
> wardly, I fulfil my duties satisfactorily in the office, not my inner
> duties, however, and every unfulfilled inner duty becomes a mis-
> fortune that never leaves. (D1 59)

Nor was Kafka's work in the insurance office the only outside activity that demanded his attention. Some of his valuable free time had to be sacrificed to supervising in a hat factory owned by his father. In 1911 he notes "the torment that the factory causes me," and details the commercial anxieties that "lead to the complete destruction of my existence, which, even apart from this, becomes more and more hedged in." (D1 201) But several years later his situation is as desperate as ever. Bluntly: "I shall not be able to write as long as I have to go to the factory," he mourns, highlighting his antipathy with a striking image:

> Immediate contact with the workaday world deprives me . . .
> of the possibility of taking a broad view of matters, just as if I
> were at the bottom of a ravine, with my head bowed down in
> addition. (D2 109)

And yet, alongside all this, more than once he expresses the
thought that he is to blame, he owes the office a full day's work.
"In the final analysis," he admits in February, 1911, "the fault
is mine, and the office has a right to make the most definite and
justified demands on me." (D1 44)  And Max Brod presents a
picture of Kafka spending long and arduous hours (overtime!)
preparing reports that were the epitome of bureaucratic minutia,
while on his desk at home an unfinished story awaited his attention.

Hence Brod's contention that "literary work was not the be-
all and end-all for Kafka, however much many passages in the
diary, if taken literally, might seem to say so."[7] On the contrary,
writes Brod, "it was life in the social community and significant
work that meant the highest goal and ideal for him."[8]

The overall picture is one of conflict and ambivalence. Objectively, there was nothing "significant" about Kafka's work with
the Institute; he was a minion, his reports could be done by anyone (as he well knew), while the story on his desk could be com-
pleted only by him. As for his father's factory, Kafka himself
reasoned that even if he could somehow fathom all the details
of its operation, "what would I have achieved?" (D1 201) Nevertheless, he reproached himself when he neglected his "duties"
there.

After 1917, when his tubercular condition was definitely es-
tablished, Kafka stopped working regularly and was able to de-
vote more time to his writing. But one of his later aphorisms is
a wry reminder of the past: "His weariness is that of the gladia-
tor after the combat; his work was the whitewashing of a corner
in a state official's office."[9]

## 2 WOMEN AND MARRIAGE

Kafka's attitude towards women was extremely ambivalent. He easily made friends with them, but he feared them too. "Women are snares," he is quoted as saying, "which lie in wait for men on all sides in order to drag them into the merely finite." [10]

His few sexual contacts were apparently not very successful. In July, 1916, he writes:

> I have never yet been intimate with a woman apart from that time in Zuckmantel. And then again with the Swiss girl in Riva. The first was a woman, and I was ignorant; the second a child, and I was utterly confused. (D2 159)

Another diary entry in 1916 suggests he knew the compulsion (and transience) of "anima fascinations" [11] :

> What a muddle I've been in with girls, in spite of all my head-aches, insomnia, gray hair, despair. Let me count them: there have been at least six since the summer. I can't resist, my tongue is fairly torn from my mouth if I don't give in and ad-mire anyone who is admirable and love her until admiration is exhausted. (D2 154)

It is possible Kafka was impotent. "What have you done with your gift of sex?" he asks himself in January, 1922. "It was a failure, in the end that is all that they will say." (D2 203) Max Brod mentions occasional visits to brothels, but more often Kafka simply toyed with the idea:

> I intentionally walk through streets where there are whores. Walking past them excites me, the remote but nevertheless ex-istent possibility of going with one. (D1 309)

In a letter written late in his life, Kafka recounted his first sexual experience with a woman (a prostitute). Of it, he said he was relieved that "the whole experience hadn't been *more* horrible, *more* obscene." [12] On the whole, his attitude towards sex seems to be summed up in one sentence: "Coitus as punishment for the happiness of being together." (D1 296)

Of marriage, however, Kafka had the highest conception. "There is no one here who understands me in my entirety," runs a typical diary entry. "To have someone possessed of such understanding, a wife perhaps, would mean to have support from every side, to have God." (D2 126) In the famous *Letter to His Father*, written in 1920, when Kafka was 37 years old, he writes:

> Marrying, founding a family, accepting all the children that come, supporting them in this insecure world and even guiding them a little as well, is, I am convinced, the utmost a human being can succeed in doing at all. [13]

And in 1922:

> The infinite, deep, warm, saving happiness of sitting beside the cradle of one's child opposite its mother.
>
> There is in it also something of this feeling: matters no longer rest with you, unless you wish it so. In contrast, this feeling of those who have no children: it perpetually rests with you, whether you will or no, every moment to the end, every nerve-wracking moment, it perpetually rests with you, and without result. Sisyphus was a bachelor. (D2 204-205)

It is clear that Kafka's art, the progeny he bred in solitude, was not, in itself, enough. Yet every attempt to marry and "found a family" was frustrated by inner conflicts.

For five years Kafka was on the verge of marrying a young Berlin girl, Felice Bauer. He met her in August, 1912. It was a tormenting affair for both parties, marked by extreme mood swings. In June, 1914: "Convinced that I need F." (D2 62) In July, 1916: "Impossible to live with F." (D2 157) They were engaged, the engagement broken, engaged again, and again broken. In August,

1913, he writes to Max Brod: "I love her, as far as I am capable of that, but my love is buried almost to suffocation under fear and self-reproaches." [14] And to the girl in October, 1916:

> You belong to me, I have taken you to myself. I can't believe that in any fairy story any woman was more often and more desperately fought for, than you were in me.[15]

But it was all to no avail; their relationship was decisively ended (by Kafka, and with some sense of relief) in December, 1917, when his tuberculosis was diagnosed. One of his last references to her in his diary sums it all up in one line: "The whips with which we lash each other have put forth many knots these five years." (D2 187)

Another two years were spent in soul-searchings over the possibility of life with Milena Jesenska, the woman who translated his early short stories into Czech. They actually met only twice, but Kafka wrote her hundreds of letters — an orgy of despair, bliss, self-laceration, and self-humiliation. (Max Brod: "To my mind they belong among the most significant love-letters of all time."[16]) Milena, although unhappily married, could not bring herself to leave her husband. Kafka, victimized by his usual inner insecurity, would settle for nothing less. Their letter-romance died soon after he wrote her:

> The possibility of a shared life which we thought we had in Vienna, does not exist, under no conditions, it didn't even exist then, I had looked "over my fence," had just held on to the top with my hands, then I fell back again with lacerated hands. There are of course other possibilities of sharing, the world's full of possibilities, but I don't know them yet.[17]

These two major failures, and several shorter affairs, confirmed Kafka in the belief that he was "mentally incapable of marrying":

> This manifests itself in the fact that from the moment I make up my mind to marry I can no longer sleep, my head burns day and night, life can no longer be called life, I stagger about in despair.[18]

In December, 1911, long before it became clear that he would never marry, Kafka expressed his intense longing for children, and unwittingly forecast his own fate:

> An unfortunate man, one who is condemned to have no chil-
> dren, is terribly imprisoned in his own misfortune. Nowhere
> a hope for revival, for help from luckier stars. He must live his
> life afflicted by his misfortune, and when its circle is ended
> must resign himself to it and not start out again to see whether,
> on a longer path, under other circumstances of body and time,
> the misfortune which he has suffered could disappear or even
> produce something good.[19] (D1 200)

Only in the last year of his life did Kafka find some degree of shared contentment with a woman. That was with Dora Dymant, a young girl barely half his age. Kafka met her while on holiday in the summer of 1923 in Müritz, the Baltic seaside resort. Captivated, he returned to Prague, cut all his ties, and went to live with her in Berlin. She was at his side when his health finally collapsed and he died on June 3, 1924.

## 3 FAMILY

Kafka's relationship with his parents was no consolation for the lack of a family of his own. Although he lived with his mother and father almost all his life, he felt "more strange than a stranger." (D1 299) He kept to himself, avoiding the social life of his parents. He resented any demands on his time, the least interference in his affairs. In August, 1913, he writes:

> I have not spoken an average of twenty words a day to my
> mother these last years, hardly ever said hello to my father. . . .
> Everything that is not literature bores me and I hate it, for it
> disturbs me or delays me, if only because I think it does. I lack
> all aptitude for family life except, at best, as an observer. I
> have no family feeling and visitors make me almost feel as
> though I were maliciously being attacked. (D1 299-300)

His father, a self-made businessman, had no appreciation of Kafka's "sensitive" nature or his literary talent. In the *Letter to His Father*, Kafka writes that his father's "method of upbringing" had saddled him with "a general load of fear, weakness and self-contempt,"[20] which arrested his development not only with regard to marriage — described by Kafka as his "most large-scale and hopeful attempt to escape"[21] — but in every sphere of life:

> Where I lived I was an outcast, condemned, defeated, and al-
> though I struggled my utmost to flee elsewhere, it was labour
> in vain, because I was trying to do something that was impos-
> sible, that was beyond my strength except for a few insignifi-
> cant exceptions.[22]

Although Kafka had scant respect for his father's material values, he desperately wanted his approval: "My opinion of myself depended more on you than on anything else, such as, for example, on any outward success."[23] A kind word from his father, a blessing on his efforts in any field, would, thought Kafka, have strengthened him to face a hostile world. Instead:

> In front of you I lost my self-confidence and exchanged it for an infinite sense of guilt. In the recollection of this infinity I once wrote about someone, quite truly, "He is afraid the shame will even live on after him."[24]

Nor was his mother any help:

> She considers me a healthy young man who suffers a little from the notion that he is ill. This notion will disappear by itself with time; marriage, of course, and having children would put an end to it best of all. Then my interest in literature would also be reduced to the degree that is perhaps necessary for an educated man.  (D1 184-185)

In Kafka's view, she was in league with his father, they formed a common bond against him. During his childhood, his mother left the house in the morning to help her husband in the business. In the evenings, his father monopolized her time in playing cards.

Photographs of Kafka's mother show a strong, determined, square-cut face and a stalwart figure — indeed, a mannish woman, whose activities and opinions immediately suggest the "animus woman."[25] "How furious I am with my mother," writes Kafka in December, 1913. "I need only begin to talk to her and I am irritated, almost scream." (D1 317) In October, 1916: "Father from one side, mother from the other, have inevitably almost broken my spirit." (D2 168) And in the letter to his father, he describes his mother as having "unconsciously played the role of beater during a hunt."[26] That is to say, he saw his mother flushing him out into the open so that his father could finish him off.

Kafka never became close to his parents, and of his three younger sisters he was only fond of Ottilie (the youngest and nine years his junior). Several times he moved out and tried to manage completely on his own, but these attempts never amounted to much;

intolerable as it was to live at home, it was even more unbearable to be on his own. "Living alone," he notes in July, 1914, "ends only with punishment." (D2 75)

The unsatisfactory nature of Kafka's home life is strikingly expressed in a conversation he had with Gustav Janouch, a young poet whose father worked in the same insurance office as Kafka. Janouch, who had regular talks with Kafka for two years (1920-1922), on subjects ranging from religion to art and from dreams to reality, quotes Kafka:

> I am now going home. But it only looks as if I were. In reality, I mount into a prison specially constructed for myself, which is all the harsher because it looks like a perfectly ordinary bourgeois home and — except for myself — no one would recognize it as a prison. For that reason, every attempt at escape is useless. One cannot break one's chains when there are no chains to be seen.[27]

# 4 TWO WORLDS

"Solitude is powerful beyond anything else," runs one of
Kafka's diary fragments, "and drives one back to people. Naturally, you then attempt to find new ways, ways seemingly less
painful but in reality simply not yet known." (D2 81) Kafka's
own search for "ways seemingly less painful," every attempt to
relate himself happily and productively to "life in the social community," was unsuccessful.

Denied trust and understanding in the home, defeated in his
ambition to marry and have children, Kafka was left with only
himself and his writing. In January, 1922, acknowledging his failures, Kafka notes in his diary:

> There is an artificial, miserable substitute for everything, for
> forebears, marriage and heirs. Feverishly you contrive these
> substitutes, and if the fever has not already destroyed you, the
> hopelessness of the substitutes will. (D2 207)

Intent on exploring and portraying what he called his "dreamlike inner life," (D2 77) Kafka yet yearned for a more "normal"
life, a more "productive" existence in the real world of everyday
life. Indeed, there is abundant evidence in the diaries and elsewhere to support Max Brod's contention that two opposite ten-
dencies fought for supremacy in Kafka: "the longing for loneliness and the will to be sociable."[28] In Kafka's own view, he existed in a kind of no-man's land:

> I have seldom, very seldom crossed this borderland between
> loneliness and fellowship, I have even been settled there longer
> than in loneliness itself. What a fine bustling place was Robinson
> Crusoe's island in comparison! (D2 198)

Further, as mentioned above, Brod insists that "the tendency

to loneliness . . . he disapproved of, and it was life in the social
community and significant work that meant the highest goal and
ideal for him."[29] But certainly the ambivalence was there, and
it is nowhere more poignantly expressed than in one of his short
pieces called "The Street Window":

> Whoever leads a solitary life, and yet now and then wants to
> attach himself somewhere; whoever, according to changes in the
> time of day, the weather, the state of his business and the like,
> suddenly wishes to see any arm at all to which he might cling —
> he will not be able to manage for long without a window look-
> ing on to the street.[30]

It is this conflict that gives a noticeably *wistful* quality to
Kafka's expressions of his isolation — a distinct longing that it
could be otherwise. "The attraction of the human world is so
immense," he mourns in January, 1922, "in an instant it can make
one forget everything," and continues:

> Yet the attraction of my world too is strong; those who love
> me love me because I am "forsaken" . . . because they sense
> that in happy moments I enjoy on another plane the freedom
> of movement completely lacking to me here. (D2 215)

Kafka's "other world" is a private, inner world, the world of
the soul, the seeker after transcendental truth. To this world
Kafka devoted his creative energies. "I get my principal nourish-
ment from other roots in other climes," he declares. "These roots
too are sorry ones, but nevertheless," he adds — and considering
his ambivalence it is a hopeful addition — "better able to sustain
life." (D2 215)

Among a list of aphorisms written in 1920, Kafka said that
his wish had been

> to attain a view of life (and — this was necessarily bound up
> with it — to convince others of it in writing) in which life,
> while still retaining its natural, full-bodied rise and fall, would
> simultaneously be recognized no less clearly as a nothing, a
> dream, a dim hovering.[31]

"This is far," as Nietzsche remarked, "and only the swift reach it and are delighted."[32] The evidence of Kafka's literary work is that he reached it; the evidence of a life marked with melancholy, frustration, and despair is that he was not often delighted. "If I am condemned to die," he writes in July, 1916, "then I am not only condemned to die, but also condemned to struggle until I die." (D2 161)

Thomas Mann, in his short story *Tonio Kröger*, has pinpointed this dilemma as an essential element in the modern artist's relation to society. "I love life," declares Kröger, and continues:

> We who are set apart and different do not conceive life as, like us, unusual; it is the normal, respectable, and admirable that is the kingdom of our longing: life, in all its seductive banality! That man is far from being an artist . . . who does not know a longing for the innocent, the simple and the living, for a little friendship, devotion, familiar human happiness — the gnawing, surreptitious hankering for the bliss of the commonplace.[33]

Kröger's confession is interpreted by a friend as a sign that he is "a bourgeois on the wrong path, a bourgeois *manqué*." The same might be suggested of Kafka, but it is doubtful if he could have turned the accusation into Kröger's defiant manifesto: "If anything is capable of making a poet out of a literary man, it is my bourgeois love of the human, the living and the usual."[34]

But it is no surprise to read in Brod's biography that *Tonio Kröger* was a favorite of Kafka's, for he could certainly echo Kröger's lament, namely: "I stand between two worlds. I am at home in neither, and I suffer in consequence."[35]

That is precisely the refrain that runs through Kafka's life, a near-endless lament due to the raising of hopes in both worlds, the inner and the outer.

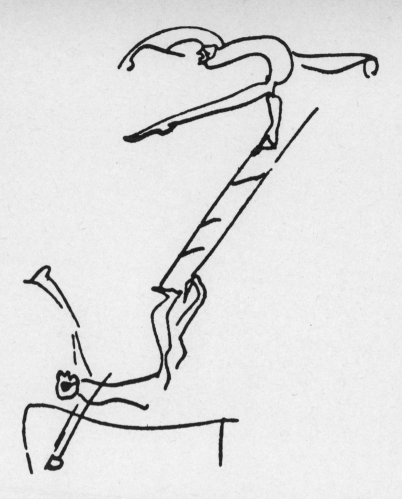

My condition is not unhappiness, but it is also not happiness, not indifference, not weakness, not fatigue, not another interest—so what is it then? That I do not know this is probably connected with my inability to write. And without knowing the reason for it, I believe I understand the latter. All those things, that is to say, those things which occur to me, occur to me not from the root up but rather only from somewhere about their middle. Let someone then attempt to seize them, let someone attempt to seize a blade of grass and hold fast to it when it begins to grow only from the middle.

There are some people who can do this, probably, Japanese jugglers, for example, who scramble up a ladder that does not rest on the ground but on the raised soles of someone half lying on the ground, and which does not lean against a wall but just goes up into the air. I cannot do this—aside from the fact that my ladder does not even have those soles at its disposal.

—Detail from a manuscript page of Kafka's *Diaries* (see text page 10)

# PART TWO:
# PSYCHOLOGICAL

# 1  CONFLICT

Kafka's complaints about his job (and the unwanted responsibilities in his father's factory) are classic expressions of frustration in an artist tied to time-consuming obligations he could better do without. The question that immediately arises is why he couldn't give them up.

It is not difficult to find reasons. Certainly, he had no independent means of support, and he would have suffered worse ordeals rather than be a financial burden on his parents, even though they could well afford it. Max Brod suggests stubbornness: ". . . a passive tenacity . . . he suffered and kept silent."[36] Kafka himself could find many reasons, for instance in his conversation in 1911 with Dr. Steiner:

> Aside from my family relationships, I could not live by literature if only, to begin with, because of the slow maturing of my work and its special character; besides, I am prevented also by my health and my character from devoting myself to what is, in the most favorable case, an uncertain life.  (D1 59)

And two years later, in a letter to his fiancée's father:

> My job is unbearable to me because it conflicts with my only desire and my only calling, which is literature. . . . You might ask why I do not give up this job and — I have no money — do not try to support myself by literary work. To this I can only make the miserable reply that I don't have the strength for it, and that, as far as I can see, I shall instead be destroyed by this job, and destroyed completely.  (D1 299)

Such reasons and excuses indicate why Kafka *didn't* give up his job, but they obscure the essential issue, namely that he *couldn't.* A psychological interpretation has to start with this

29

impasse, which is at the heart of any conflict situation. One cannot act because one doesn't know what one really wants. And not knowing what one wants means not knowing who one is.

Similarly, the focal point of Kafka's inability to marry was the conflict between being alone and living intimately with another person. His extreme sensitivity to noise, his introspective nature, the slow and arduous development of his talent — these factors and others, he reasoned, demanded a more or less ascetic life. Domesticity and conjugal interdependence, he argued, would drive him to distraction. Yet this realization did not put an end to his conflict, it merely intensified it. In February, 1914, for instance, at the height of his first abortive attempt to marry Felice Bauer, Kafka writes:

> There will certainly be no one to blame if I should kill myself. . . . F. simply happens to be the one through whom my fate is made manifest; I can't live without her and must jump [out the window], yet . . . I couldn't live with her either. (D2 20)

And in July, 1916:

> Impossible to live with F. Intolerable living with anyone. I don't regret this; I regret the impossibility for me, of not living alone. (D2 157)

Again, there were many reasons why Kafka didn't marry Felice Bauer, but only one psychological answer: he couldn't because he didn't know who he was.

In general, conflict arises when there is the possibility of, and temptation to, more than one course of action. Theoretically the options may be many. In practice, a conflict is usually between two, each of which carries its own chain of consequences; for example, husband and lover, wife and mistress, two different jobs, directions, decisions, etc. And perhaps the most painful conflicts of all are those that seem to involve a choice between "security and freedom."

When a choice exists between two incompatible options, both

of which are equally attractive, the psychological reality is that two separate personalities are involved. These may be seen as personifications of complexes.[37] Each demands satisfaction; neither will sacrifice its sovereignty. Under such conditions it is the task of the individual to hold the tension between the opposites — and bear the suffering this entails — in order to discover who he (or she) really is. To make a premature choice for one or the other will simply constellate (i.e., activate) the other side more strongly.

Two preliminary possibilities exist for resolving a conflict. You can tally up the pro's and con's on each side and reach a logically satisfying decision, or you can opt to do what you "really want," and then proceed to do what is necessary to make it possible.

There is not much to say about the first way. As Jung notes, "Anything that can be decided by reason without injurious effects can safely be left to reason."[38] The trouble is that reason alone is less likely to solve a conflict than to prolong it — as it did in Kafka's case.

Serious conflicts do not so easily disappear. They require a confrontation with the unconscious — a dialogue with the "other side." That is why, faced with an analysand who has a conflict, the analyst may ask, "But what do *you* want?" or alternatively, "What do you *want*?" These questions invariably prove disconcerting to the analysand, for if he knew what he wanted he would have no conflict. Indeed, consciously he wants both, the penny and the cake.

From a psychological point of view they are useful questions, for the first, with the accent on "you," constellates the individual ego position (as opposed to what others might want); and the second, stressing "want," constellates the feeling function (judgement, evaluation[39]). Some conflicts may be resolved in this way without further ado, that is, when the ego position coincides with, or accepts, the feeling attitude. If these are not compatible, however, and the ego refuses to "give way," then the situation remains at an impasse. That is the clinical picture of neurotic conflict, and it is the story of Kafka's life.

In July, 1913, for instance, Kafka made a "summary of all the arguments for and against my marriage":

> 1. Inability to endure life alone. . . . The connection with F. will give my existence more strength to resist.

> 2. Everything immediately gives me pause. Every joke in the comic paper, what I remember about Flaubert and Grillparzer, the sight of the nightshirts on my parents' beds, laid out for the night, Max's marriage. . . .

> 3. I must be alone a great deal. What I accomplished was only the result of being alone.

> 4. I hate everything that does not relate to literature, conversations bore me . . . to visit people bores me, the sorrows and joys of my relatives bore me to my soul. Conversations take the importance, the seriousness, the truth out of everything I think.

> 5. The fear of the connection, of passing into the other. Then I'll never be alone again.

> 6. In the past, especially, the person I am in the company of my sisters has been entirely different from the person I am in the company of other people. Fearless, powerful, surprising, moved as I otherwise am only when I write. If through the intermediation of my wife I could be like that in the presence of everyone! But then would it not be at the expense of my writing? Not that, not that!

> 7. Alone, I could perhaps some day really give up my job. Married, it will never be possible. (D1 292-293)

This list reveals much about Kafka: his pervasive ambivalence, his attitude towards sex (fearful), and his paramount concern for his writing, among others. These aspects are referred to later; here I want only to point out the disparity between his ego-ideal in favour of marriage and his apparent feelings about it. In the terms I have used above, to the question "What do *you* want?" he could reply unequivocally, "To marry"; and asked, "What do you *want*?" he would have to answer quite as definitely, "Not to marry."

That is precisely the impasse that cannot be resolved on an ego level. Just as we need relationship to others to know more about ourselves, so we need the help of the mirror of the unconscious in order to be able to reflect objectively who (or rather what) we really are.

Jung, stressing the difference between knowledge of the ego and knowledge of the Self (the personality as a whole), quotes the alchemist Gerhard Dorn: "No one can know himself unless he knows *what,* and not *who,* he is." Notes Jung:

> The distinction between "quis" [who] and "quid" [what]
> is crucial: whereas "quis" has an unmistakably personal aspect
> and refers to the ego, "quid" is neuter, predicating . . . . the
> psyche itself as the unknown, unprejudiced object that still has
> to be investigated.[40]

That is to say, what is usually thought of as "self-knowledge" is inadequate precisely because it is subjective and therefore inclined to be clouded by "blind spots" (complexes). True, objective knowledge of oneself comes through paying attention to the attitude of the unconscious — as it appears, for example, in dreams.

Now, Kafka was certainly interested in dreams in general. A dreamlike quality is characteristic of his work, and there is evidence that he incorporated some of his dreams in a modified form in his stories.[41] But he had a low opinion of psychology in general and Freudian psychoanalysis in particular. "There is no pleasure in spending any time on psychoanalysis," he wrote, "and I keep as aloof from it as I possibly can."[42] He looked upon the therapeutic claims of psychoanalysis as "an impotent error."[43] Too much psychology "nauseated" him, and he declared: "Never again psychology."[44] Kafka mocked the student of psychology as a good runner who can "in a short time and in any zigzag he likes, cover distances such as he cannot cover in any other field. One's eyes overbrim at the sight."[45] Psychology, he observed, is impatience,[46] and for Kafka this was the cardinal sin: "Because of impatience we were driven out of Paradise . . . . because of impatience we cannot return."[47]

Such strong resistance to "psychology" usually indicates the unconscious need for it; that is, something unconscious is pressing to be acknowledged, but the threatened ego brings forth whatever rationalizations and defenses are necessary to keep the unknown at bay — rather than relinquish the illusion that one is "master in one's own house." The result, in a situation like Kafka's, is to harden the ego attitude and make change next to impossible.

One consequence of Kafka's aversion to what he knew of psychology and psychoanalysis is that he never took his dreams seriously as a source of information about himself. "Almost impossible to sleep," he notes in February, 1922, "plagued by dreams [a common complaint], as if they were being scratched on me, on a stubborn material."[48] (D2 218) This suggests that his unconscious was clamouring for attention, but he "stubbornly" refused to pay heed. The same attitude is explicit in a diary entry more than ten years earlier: "When I awaken," he writes in October, 1911, "all the dreams are gathered about me, but *I am careful not to reflect on them.*" (D1 74; my italics)

This attitude puts Kafka in the company of Parsifal, the hero of the Grail legend, who when he was first confronted with the phenomenon of the Holy Grail was so overcome with awe and reverence that he failed to ask the right questions, namely: "What does all this have to do with me, what does it mean to me, about me?" To ask such questions is another way to constellate the feeling function, as opposed to wallowing in emotion. The consequence of Parsifal's emotional stupour was that the Grail (and castle) vanished, and he had to spend many long years wandering through the forest (the unconscious) before he finally came upon it again, asked the questions, and healed the wounded Fisher King. In this legend and many others, the old or wounded king is psychologically analogous to the dominant attitude of consciousness that needs to be renewed because it no longer works, it is not appropriate to a particular life situation.[49]

In these terms, Kafka's conscious attitude was "wounded," his wound manifesting in indecisiveness and the inability to resolve his conflicts. One potential source of renewal would have been his dreams.

The importance of dreams lies in the fact that they are an independent, spontaneous product of the unconscious. Thus the information they contain serves to compensate the generally one-sided attitudes of consciousness. "Compensation," writes Jung, "means *balancing, adjusting, supplementing.*"[50] Dreams have a compensatory function in the individual psyche in that they reveal aspects of the personality that are normally unconscious; they disclose unconscious motivations operating in relationships; and they reveal new points of view and new ways of dealing with conflict situations.

Among Kafka's published dreams there is one that concerns Felice Bauer. A methodical analysis of this dream can tell us a good deal about Kafka's psychology that would account for the impasse between them. Kafka recorded it in his diary on February 13, 1914, three months before their first official engagement:

> In Berlin, through the streets to her house, calm and happy
> in the knowledge that, though I haven't arrived at her house yet,
> a slight possibility of doing so exists; I shall certainly arrive
> there. I see the streets, on a white house a sign, something
> like "The Splendors of the North" (saw it in the paper yester-
> day); in my dream "Berlin W" has been added to it. Ask the way
> of an affable, red-nosed old policeman who in this instance is
> stuffed into a sort of butler's livery. Am given excessively de-
> tailed directions, he even points out the railing of a small park in
> the distance which I must keep hold of for safety's sake when
> I go past. Then advice about the trolley, the subway, etc. I
> can't follow him any longer and ask in a fright, knowing full
> well that I am underestimating the distance: "That's about half
> an hour away?" But the old man answers, "I can make it in six

minutes." What joy! Some man, a shadow, a companion, is always at my side. I don't know who it is. Really have no time
to turn around, to turn sideways. (D2 19)

Berlin is where Felice lived. The "white house" suggests deliver-
ance, salvation, the purity of the wedding dress. In alchemy lunar
whiteness is the *albedo*, associated with spirit and the Queen, the
opposite of the red King. White is also connected with snow,
surely one of "the Splendours of the North." The north has connotations of darkness, cold, winter, death, and night. In Germanic
folklore it is the abode of the gods, that is the unconscious, and
in Celtic mythology it is the place where the White Goddess of
the Moon imprisoned the dead sun-kings.

A policeman is a symbol of authority; a butler serves. Here the
two are confused and combined into a figure of derision. The
nose is a common symbol for intuition; also, being phallic in
shape, it relates to the masculine attitude. Here it is red, suggesting not only the heat of emotion but also the ravages of alcohol,
a form of spirit or Logos, which is itself associated with the thinking function. The red nose would thus indicate both some damage
to the masculinity (distorted by emotion) and an intuitive function contaminated by too much thinking.

The "excessively detailed directions" call to mind the care and
concern of a mother for her little boy. The policeman/butler,
therefore, not only lacks credibility as a figure of authority, he
functions in the dream as a servant of the Great Mother — perhaps
one of the palace eunuchs of the Moon Goddess, his red nose then
relating to the other indications of cold, north, winter, etc.

The policeman's detailed directions also imply it would take
forever to find "the way." (Kafka: "The true way . . . . seems more
designed to make people stumble than to be walked upon."[51])
But the old man says he can make it in six minutes. Six commonly
refers to relationship problems (as a commingling of the "female"
triangle, with apex down, and the "male" triangle, with apex up;
e.g., the Seal of Solomon); and also, through God's creation of

the world in six days, to trial and effort.

The "shadow companion" is everywhere familiar in dreams, mythology, and fairytales as the unconscious, other side of the personality, the friend and ally the protagonist ignores at his or her peril, for this companion is invariably the key to redemption or success. In the Babylonian *Epic of Gilgamesh*, it is the nature-man Enkidu (two-thirds animal and one-third human) who helps King Gilgamesh (one-third human and two-thirds divine) in his fight against the Great Mother Ishtar. Together the two make a whole (equally animal, human, divine).

At the time of this dream Kafka was plagued by doubts about Felice's affection for him. As he notes in his diary a few days later: "I often had forebodings, and fears . . . that F. did not love me very much." (D2 25) In contrast to his conscious indecision and inability to act, the message of the dream is compensatory: "I haven't arrived at her house yet," but "I shall certainly arrive there" (i.e., marry her) — if he makes the effort to create a new world, so to speak, which would be the effect of a change in attitude.

More important, however, is the symbolism associated with the "Splendours of the North" and the policeman/butler, for the suggestion is that unconsciously Kafka pictured Felice as a kind of Valkyrie from the north who would lead him to death. This is what was behind his inability to commit himself to a relationship he apparently valued so highly: an unconscious fear of the devouring mother. This is consistent with Kafka's remark to Gustav Janouch, quoted earlier, that "women are snares which lie in wait for men on all sides . . ." It is a typical fear of the *puer*, and behind it lies an unresolved mother-complex that regularly manifests in difficulties with inter-personal commitment.

As in the dream, Kafka's plans to marry always foundered on the approach — he lost his way. The policeman/butler is a personification of his ineffectual masculinity; the directions confuse rather than enlighten him, precisely because they derive from the mother-complex. His dependence in the dream on the directions of the policeman (the mother-messenger) shows his inability to function forthrightly, as a man — because he does not know what he wants. Indeed, the situation is similar to that in the fairytale "The Virgin Czar," where the Baba Yaga (witch) asks the hero, "My child, are you going voluntarily or involuntarily?" As von Franz indicates:

> This is a trick of the devouring mother's animus . . . . it is a
> trick of the mother-complex to put a philosophical ques-
> tion at just the moment when *action* is needed.[52]

What this looked like in reality, in Kafka's case, was the endless lists he compiled "for and against" his marriage — instead of getting on with it. (In the fairytale, the hero's appropriate response is: "Shut up and make my supper!")

It is interesting to see that help in solving his dilemma, his conflict, is, in the dream, right at hand — the "shadow companion" who walks at his side. What might he want? Does he know the way? Psychologically, the shadow personifies all those qualities, both positive and negative, that are not part of consciousness. To assimilate them is one way for the *puer* to depotentiate the mother-complex which holds him in thrall.

But Kafka, alas, had "no time to turn around, to turn sideways" — impatience, what he himself called "the cardinal sin" — just as he did not reflect on his dreams, did not ask the crucial question: "What does this mean to me?"

*

Jung, when commenting on the psychology of conflict situations, was fond of referring to the parable of Buridan's ass, the donkey who starved to death between two piles of hay because he couldn't make a choice. (Starving to death is an apt image for the feeling of being cut off from life, one of Kafka's many complaints and a theme he explored brilliantly in "A Hunger Artist".) In *Two Essays,* Jung writes:

The important thing was not whether the bundle on the right
or the one on the left was the better, or which one he ought
to start eating, but what he wanted in the depths of his being —
which did he feel pushed towards? The ass wanted the object
to make up his mind for him. [Kafka: "I remain alone, unless F.
will still have me after all." (D2 18)]

What is it, at this moment and in this individual, that represents the natural urge of life? That is the question.[53]

In the case of Kafka's job/writing conflict, the answer would
seem to be unequivocal. "It is easy to recognize a concentration
in me of all my forces on writing," he observes in January, 1912,
"the most productive direction for my being to take," a direction
"now interfered with only by the office, but that interferes with
it completely." (D1 211)  Yet he continued to work and he continued to complain. What, then, did he really want?

A teleological reason as to why he continued in the impasse
may be found in an earlier reference by Jung to Buridan's ass.
"I often use that example with my patients," says Jung in *The
Vision Seminars,* "and you can imagine why."

For what was the real reason that the ass acted so strangely? . . .
It was because he did not want either, there was something
more important to him. What was that?

*Answer:* To die.

*Dr. Jung:* Exactly. So he died. He committed suicide.[54]

Similarly, something in Kafka (the Self?) wanted a death — not,
surely, his physical death, but the death of his ego attitude. *"Die
nature verlangt einen Tod,"* writes Goethe — "Nature demands a
death."[55] For the death of the inappropriate ego attitude (the
"old or wounded king") is the *sine qua non* of renewal, transformation.

"A real solution" to conflict, writes Jung, "comes only from
within, and then only because the patient has been brought to a
different attitude."[56] Conflicts must be solved on a level of char-

acter where "the opposites" are taken sufficiently into account, "and this again is possible only through a change of character. . . . In such cases external solutions are worse than none at all."[57]

"Only what is really oneself," writes Jung, "has the power to heal."[58] And what that is can only be discovered through holding the tension between the opposites until a third — the *tertium non datur*, the third not logically given, the totally unexpected — manifests. This "third" (called by Jung the transcendent function) represents the creative intervention and guidance of the Self, the archetype of wholeness, which functions in the psyche as a self-regulating centre.

Without a fundamental change of attitude, then, Kafka's conflicts were inherently insoluble. At bottom they were the result of a disparity between his ego ideals and his personal limitations. In psychological terms, they were symptomatic of a split between ego and shadow, and such a split is irreparable so long as the conflict remains in the head, that is, between consciously conflicting opposites.

As usual, Kafka knew this too. "The bony structure of his own forehead blocks his way," runs one of his aphorisms, "he batters himself bloody against his own forehead."[59]

The tension involved in the conflict between ego and shadow is commonly experienced as a kind of crucifixion. This symbolizes the suffering involved in differentiating the opposites and learning to live with them. Writes Jung:

> Nobody who finds himself on the road to wholeness can escape that characteristic suspension which is the meaning of crucifixion. For he will infallibly run into things that thwart and "cross" him: first, the thing he has no wish to be (the shadow); second, the thing he is not (the "other," the individual reality of the "You"); and third, his psychic non-ego (the collective unconscious).[60]

Kafka had his own inimitable ways to describe this. For instance, he once sent a drawing to Milena with this description:

> So that you can see something of my "occupations," I'm enclos-
> ing a drawing. There are four poles, through the two middle ones
> are driven rods to which the hands of the "delinquent" are fas-
> tened; through the two outer poles rods are driven for the feet.
> After the man has been bound in this way the rods are slowly
> drawn outwards until the man is torn apart in the middle.[61]

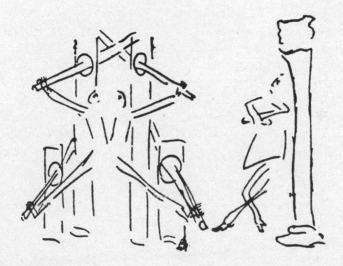

And in one of his prose fragments the same motif appears in
rather more intellectual terms:

> He is a free and secure citizen of the world, for he is fettered
> to a chain which is long enough to give him the freedom of
> all earthly space, and yet only so long that nothing can drag
> him past the frontiers of the world. But simultaneously he is a
> free and secure citizen of heaven as well, for he is also fettered
> by a similarly designed heavenly chain. So that if he heads, say,
> for the earth, his heavenly collar throttles him, and if he heads
> for Heaven, his earthly one does the same.[62]

These images are striking expressions of the way in which conflict can tear one asunder. Existentially, the experience is inseparable from suffering. Teleologically, in terms of what Jung has
called the individuation process, the conscious awareness of conflict is an opportunity to grow up, to heal the ego-shadow split.

Life always involves the collision between conflicting obligations. The realization and acceptance of conflict as the unavoidable fabric of life is, paradoxically, the only escape from the
cross. For Kafka — as for anyone else — "fettered" between
Christ-like ideals and the inescapable facts of physical existence,
the solution necessarily involves humility, the acknowledgement
of ego limitations. Indeed, the cross, symbol of the crucifixion
as well as much else (including resurrection) is also a form of
the mandala, a quaternity representing wholeness. [63]

In practical terms, the ego-shadow split is alleviated through
the development of the feeling function, for it is feeling that de-
termines the value of the opposites involved in any conflict situation. This process of differentiating and evaluating the opposites
goes hand in hand with a harmonious cooperation between the
principles of masculinity and femininity, which, while polar opposites, are yet complementary.

When the male ego persists in acting without the cooperation
of the feminine (personified as the anima, the man's inner *vis-a-
vis*), the result is inevitably frustration, due to the hardening of
consciousness. The *I Ching,* that ancient Chinese book of wisdom,
is instructive on this point. "If the superior man undertakes something and tries to lead," reads Hexagram 2 (The Receptive), "he
goes astray; But if he follows, he finds guidance." [64] This means
that a man has to follow his feelings.

It is through becoming aware of and following his feelings that
a man wins the anima away from the shadow (that is, differentiates her from other contents of the unconscious). But he has to
keep his head, he can't follow blindly. Before he follows, there-

fore, he must have a firm ego standpoint — he must know "where he stands."

What is required, again, is a dialogue with "the other side," in this case moods and emotions. This active process of paying attention to how he experiences himself is the way in which a man differentiates himself from the collective, and thereby discovers priceless elements of his own essential nature. The aim of the individuation process is not to overcome one's psychology, but to become familiar with it — and this in itself leads to a change in attitude towards oneself, as well as others.

The process is tantamount to "impregnating" the anima. And just as in reality every act of intercourse does not result in a child, so must the anima be ravished, so to speak, time and time again before she conceives. What she bears, metaphorically, is the long-awaited new attitude. (This new attitude, an "experiential realization," is frequently symbolized in dreams by an anima figure actually giving birth — as the eruption into consciousness of a hitherto unconscious content.)

In Kafka's case, although he was introspective to an excruciating degree, his soul-searching did not penetrate beneath the surface. Thus his anima, his inner woman, remained moody and capricious — reflected in what Kafka experienced as "not death, alas, but the endless torment of dying." (D2 77)  And his shadow, a potential source of help, was ignored.

Kafka was psychologically naive, in that he did not take the unconscious seriously. Under these circumstances, with no "Archimedean point" from which to objectively view his own personality, his conflicts were bound to remain in his head and therefore insoluble. The overall result, in psychological terms, is that for most of his life Kafka was at the mercy of his complexes; instead of having a relationship to them — a relationship determined by a conscious, male ego standpoint — he was possessed by them.

On the other hand, Kafka had something right from the beginning that many neurotics do not have — and in analysis are forced to develop — and that is a *container*. By this I mean that he contained his conflicts in himself, he did not spread his suffering around; he did not, in the language of group therapy, "let it all hang out."

We know from Max Brod that Kafka gave virtually no hint to others of his inner turmoils. Describing the difference between Kafka as his friends knew him, and the image of Kafka one gets from his writings, Brod comments as follows:

> I have experienced over and over again that admirers of Kafka who know him only from his books have a completely false picture of him. They think he must have made a sad, even desperate impression in company too. The opposite is the case. One felt well when one was with him. The richness of his thoughts, which he generally uttered in a cheerful tone, made him, to put it on the lowest level, one of the most amusing of men I have ever met, in spite of his shyness, in spite of his quietness. . . . He could be enthusiastic and carried away. There was no end to our joking and laughing — he liked a good, hearty laugh, and knew how to make his friends laugh too. . . . He was a wonderfully helpful friend. It was only in his own case that he was perplexed, helpless — an impression that, owing to his self-controlled bearing, one did not get in personal contact with him except in rare, extreme cases, but one which is undoubtedly deepened, all the same, when one reads his diary. The fact that from his books, and above all from his diary, such a totally different, much more depressing, picture may be drawn than when it is corrected and supplemented by the impressions one can add from having lived with him day by day — that is one of the reasons that persuaded me to write these memoirs.[65]

Whatever else these remarks say about Kafka, one implication is that he was self-contained in spite of the inner pressure. "He suffered," as Brod writes elsewhere, "and kept silent," describing this trait of Kafka's as "perhaps the fatal weakness of his life."[66] My feeling, on the contrary, is that it was a saving grace.

The analogy in alchemy is the *vas Hermetis*, the hermetic vessel that must be kept closed in order to allow the contents to transform through the application of heat that cannot escape. Psychologically this means not to dissipate the heat of the inner fire by acting out one's emotions, and not to contaminate one's surroundings by imposing one's unconsciousness, including projections, on other people.

The same principle is involved in analysis, where it is a matter of respecting what is called the *temenos*, a Greek word meaning "sacred place," used to describe the sacred quality of the relationship that arises between analyst and analysand. In the analytical relationship the *temenos*, as container, is a place where the gods may safely play in an atmosphere of mutual trust and respect which is essentially private and immune to disturbing influences from the outside, profane world. (This is also the function, psychologically, of the medical Hippocratic Oath.)

In a slightly different sense, but with a similar effect, it seems to me that Kafka's container was his writing, and in particular his diary. With this in mind it is possible that Kafka's literary work possessed for him a primarily therapeutic function; it was the medium through which he exteriorized his dilemmas and thus to a certain extent obtained some perspective on them. The reluctance with which he permitted publication during his lifetime, and the fact that he left instructions for all his manuscripts to be destroyed, support this view. "My last request," wrote Kafka to Max Brod,

> is that all the writings I may leave behind me (in bookcases and drawers, in my rooms, in the office, or wherever any of them may have got to); everything in notebooks, manuscript, sheets and letters, whether my own or other people's; everything finished or in rough draft which you may have in your possession or can get hold of in my name — shall be burned at once unread.[67]

My concern here is not with why Max Brod disregarded such explicit instructions, but with why Kafka gave them. And my suggestion is that they represent an urge, albeit unconscious, to protect his personal *temenos* even after his death.

Within his vessel, his personal *temenos*, Kafka stewed for most of his life. Although he did not consciously resolve his conflicts, he did hold the tension, he did not give in; that is, he did not give up his writing nor did he renounce his high ideals about "life in the social community." Nor did he kill himself, though several times he toyed with the idea — on one occasion resisting because "by staying alive I should interrupt my writing less . . . than by dying."[68]

A remark of Nietzsche's springs to mind: "The only thing that can prove whether one has worth or not — that one holds out."[69] The same idea is expressed by Jung in different words:

> The opus [the individuation process] consists of three parts: insight, endurance, and action. Psychology is needed only in the first part, but in the second and third parts moral strength plays the predominant role.[70]

"Insight, endurance, and action." Kafka had plenty of insights, and his endurance was remarkable, but he was unable to *act*. However, there is much evidence from friends and associates that attest to Kafka's moral strength, and it would seem that in the long run this was decisive in terms of his ability to hold the tension generated by his conflicts, until at last there was a change in his attitude that made possible a concrete change in his life situation. In psychological terms, the "third," the transcendent function, did finally manifest. Furthermore, it was as Jung describes it: "a subjective experience . . . of a religious order,"[71] "an experience of the *numinosum*,"[72] "an autonomous psychic happening."[73]

But that did not happen until near the end of Kafka's short life. In the meantime, he continued the daily, unremitting struggle to reconcile the demands of his inner world with the desire to lead a more "productive" existence in the real world of everyday life. And if in retrospect the tension between Kafka's various opposites may be seen as the stimulus to some of his best writing, that was hardly a consolation to him at the time. As he notes in September, 1917:

> Have never understood how it is possible for almost everyone
> who writes to objectify his sufferings in the very midst of under-
> going them; thus I, for example, in all likelihood with my head
> still smarting from unhappiness, sit down and write to someone:
> I am unhappy. Yes, I can even go beyond that and with as many
> flourishes as I have the talent for, all of which seem to have
> nothing to do with my unhappiness, ring simple, or contrapun-
> tal, or a whole orchestration of changes on my theme. And it
> is not a lie, and it does not still my pain. (D2 184)

## 2 THE CHTHONIC SHADOW

In clinical terms, Kafka's condition was one of neurotic depression. His symptoms were depressive moods, indecision, conflict, ambivalence, lack of energy, insomnia, and chronic headaches, among others. A diary entry in October, 1921, when Kafka was 38 years old, describes how it felt:

> I don't believe people exist whose inner plight resembles mine;
> still, it is possible for me to imagine such people — but that
> the secret raven forever flaps about their heads as it does about
> mine, even to imagine that is impossible. (D2 195)

In alchemy, the raven is a symbol for the *nigredo*, which corresponds psychologically to the shadow, or rather the encounter with the shadow, which manifests initially as depression. "The principle of the art," according to one alchemical text, "is the raven, who flies without wings in the blackness of the night and in the brightness of the day."[74] Jung comments:

> The alchemists called their *nigredo* melancholia, "a black
> blacker than black," night, an affliction of the soul, confusion,
> etc., or, more pointedly, the "black raven."[75]

The alchemists' raven "flies without wings," so in a sense it is grounded. Kafka's raven flaps about his head (perhaps to call attention to itself), forever off the ground. His image of the "secret raven," then, suggests that his chthonic shadow — that portion of a man's psyche which roots him to the earth and draws new strength from below — which ought to bring him down to earth, is up in the air.

A similar conclusion emerges when we look closely at a dream he had ten years earlier, at the age of 28:

I dreamed today of a donkey that looked like a greyhound,
it was very cautious in its movements. I looked at it closely
because I was aware how unusual a phenomenon it was, but
remember only that its narrow human feet could not please
me because of their length and uniformity. I offered it a
bunch of fresh, dark-green cypress leaves which I had just
received from an old Zürich lady (it all took place in
Zürich), it did not want it, just sniffed at it; but then, when
I left the cypress on a table, it devoured it so completely that
only a scarcely recognizable kernel resembling a chestnut
was left. Later there was talk that this donkey had never yet
gone on all fours but always held itself erect like a human
being and showed its silvery shining breast and its little
belly. (D1 119)

The ass is well known as a symbol of lasciviousness. As an
animal belonging to the crowd of Dionysus, it was associated
with the Dionysian ecstasy, sexuality, and drunkenness. In the
Egyptian religion, the ass was a symbol of the god Set, who personified the principles of murder, lying, and brutality — evil par
excellence, the counterpart of the great god-man Osiris. In as-
trology, the ass is attributed to Saturn and considered to have
the qualities of that planet: drivenness, creative depression and
despair, heaviness, suffering, imprisonment, helplessness, de-
humanization.[76]

On the other hand, the ass is also associated with Christ, both
through Christ's earlier identification with Dionysus, and the
fact that he rode a donkey into Jerusalem. Also the birth of
Christ was witnessed by an ass. Hence in the Middle Ages the ass
was represented as the carrier animal of Christianity.

The ass is thus a complex symbol pointing both ways: up, to
the Christlike nature of man, and down, to his chthonic, earthy,
sexual instinct.

Here, however, we have an ass that "looked like a greyhound,"
a lean, slim dog that runs so fast it barely touches the ground.

For seven thousand years greyhounds have been bred for their
speed. King Solomon spoke of greyhounds as animals that "go
well and are comely in going." They were originally taught to
race across the Egyptian desert after game (jackals, gazelles, and
hares) until their prey was exhausted, then drag them down.
According to a fourteenth-century writer, the greyhound should
be "headed like a snake, footed like a cat, tailed like a rat."
Their only requirement is speed, for they do not track prey, but
pursue it by sight.[77]

This suggests that the chthonic drive symbolized by the ass is
too light and insubstantial, too spiritual ("windy"). In other
words, where there should be body there is too much spirit.

The fact that the ass/greyhound has "narrow human feet"
suggests a humanizing of the instinct. This is necessary and de-
sirable at some point, but the instinct can only be properly
"tamed" through first accepting it for what it is: bare-assed,
stubborn, and brutish — just as Lucius, in Apuleius' story *The
Golden Ass,* had to live out his ass nature (lust, concupiscence)
before he could be transformed by eating the roses of Isis. The
donkey here, however, "had never yet gone on all fours but always held itself erect like a human being . . ." — an indication
that the dreamer had never accepted the animality symbolized
by the ass. Its "silvery shining breast" points to a feminization
of the instinct that is entirely inappropriate in a man; psychologically, this indicates a contamination of shadow and anima.

The ass/greyhound is a creature that could not be met with in
reality. Such bastard animal forms in dreams, according to von
Franz, show that it is not an instinctive drive which wants to
find expression, but an essentially *symbolic* content inaccessible
to consciousness:

> If the unconscious wants to bring up a psychological content
> which is still so far away from consciousness that it can only be
> represented by making a *mixtum compositum* of many animal

drives . . . that shows that it is a content for which consciousness has not as yet any organ of reception.[78]

This would mean that here it is not the sex drive per se that has
to be assimilated by consciousness, but rather the symbolic significance of the *coincidentia oppositorum* represented by the
opposites ass and greyhound; i.e., the contamination of body
and spirit.

The cypress is a graveyard tree, symbolic of death and mourn-
ing, and, because of its evergreen leaves and incorruptible resin, a
symbol also of resurrection (rebirth, life after death); that is to
say, a symbol both marking death and celebrating everlasting
life (as does the tombstone). In ancient China, to eat grains of
cypress was supposed to give long life because these grains are
rich in *yang* substance (maleness).[79]

The fresh green leaves are given to the dream-ego by "an old
Zürich lady." This might actually refer to some encounter in
reality (since Kafka had been to Zürich two months previously),
but symbolically she would be what is experienced in a man's
psyche as "the old wise woman," broadly speaking the "wisdom
of nature."[80] She knows the chthonic ass requires this life food
(to compensate a conscious ascetic attitude), for like Balaam's
ass in the Old Testament, who saw the angel when Balaam did
not (Numbers 22:23), this chthonic animal drive has an intel-
ligence valuable in itself, the complement of the intellect of consciousness.

The donkey in the dream doesn't eat while it is being observed — just as an instinct may not function properly when it
is too closely watched. This is especially true of the sex instinct,
and can be the result of too much self-analysis (leading to self-
consciousness). It is as if nature were to rebel against the ego
overstepping its boundaries, and arrogating to itself control over
something that is intrinsically autonomous. The balance between
instinct and consciousness is a delicate one, easily disturbed. As

Jung notes: "Too much of the animal distorts the civilized man, too much civilization makes sick animals."[81]

But the ass is certainly hungry, for when left alone he "devours" the cypress leaves, leaving only "a kernel resembling a chestnut."

The kernel may refer to the core, the centre, the mystery of life. In the Middle Ages the nut was looked upon as an image of Christ; like the egg, it is a latent anticipation of the Self. Here the ass as sexual libido and a symbol for Christ come together; for after sex there is always something left over — libido (that is, psychic energy in general) that demands to be used in another way: creatively, religiously. The voracious appetite of the ass indicates that it is not being fed properly, a situation that would inevitably inhibit the realization of either the sensual or the divine aspect of the instinct.

How does this dream relate to Kafka? What does it say about him? Why did he have it?

The saturnine characteristics associated with the ass certainly apply to him: he was driven (as we know from his compulsion to write); he was depressed; he knew despair, felt heavy and helpless; he suffered, and experienced his life as a prison. Why? Well, the psychological reality is that whatever potential one has within oneself but does not live grows against one, it becomes negative. And that is what seems to have happened to Kafka; he suppressed his "ass" nature, he didn't give it a chance to live. Returning to the analogy of Buridan's ass, Kafka's ass got no hay at all.

We know that Kafka was almost morbidly preoccupied with his body. In 1910, seven years before his tuberculosis was diagnosed, he writes of the "despair over my body and over a future with this body." (D1 11) Other diary entries refer to his "shabby chest," his "weak heart" and "senile strength," and his body as one "picked up in a lumber room." (D1 14, 160, 162) He worried constantly about his health. His diaries record a wide range of ailments, including constipation, indigestion, insomnia, falling hair, headaches, and curvature of the spine. Max Brod testifies that "every imperfection of the body tormented him, even, for example, scurf [dandruff] , or constipation, or a toe that was not properly formed."[82]

Hypochondria, it may be noted, is a typical compensatory symptom of the *puer* — particularly one with an inferior sensation function, as Kafka almost certainly had — in that it forces him to pay attention to bodily reality. Kafka's pencil drawings (unconscious scribbles), on the other hand, frequently show tall, skinny, rather "airy" (or "windy") figures completely lacking in substance (see next page) — an accusation he often levelled at himself.

In appearance, Kafka actually was tall and thin — over six feet, weighing 55 kilos (about 120 pounds) in 1922. He was good-looking, with regular features, dark eyes and hair. Until his death he retained a youthful appearance; at forty, according to reports, he looked more like a man in his early twenties. One of his friends speaks of Kafka's quality of "childlike naivité." (Both these characteristics point to *puer* psychology.) He was a vegetarian, tee-total, took cold showers, walked, swam, rode, and had a life-long interest in health diets and nature cures. Yet he was sickly, and blamed only himself; for instance in October, 1921:

> I never learned anything useful and — the two are connected — have allowed myself to become a physical wreck . . . It is astounding how I have systematically destroyed myself in the course of the years, it was like a slowly widening breach in a dam, a purposeful action. (D2 194-195)

In addition, Kafka's attitude towards sex was puritanical. "Love always appears hand in hand with filth," he said to Gustav Janouch. "Only the will of the loved one can divide the love from the filth."[83] And to Milena:"I'm dirty, Milena, infinitely dirty, which is why I make so much fuss about purity."[84]

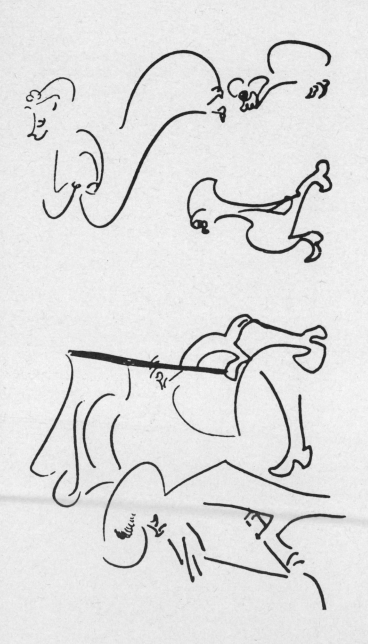

Kafka Sketch (undated)

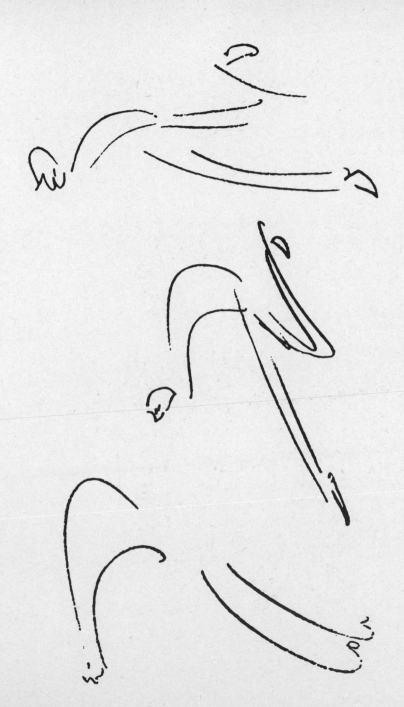

Kafka Sketch (undated)

I have already mentioned Kafka's views on some of his early sex experiences, and noted his remarkable statement about intercourse: "Coitus as punishment for the happiness of being together." And Brod recalls that Kafka "never told a dirty story or even stood for one being told in his presence."[85] There is also the following diary entry in 1922, combining self-loathing with disgust:

> All that he deserves is the dirty unknown old woman with shrunken thighs who drains his semen in an instant, pockets the money and hurries off to the next room where another customer is already waiting for her. (D2 227)

Perhaps nowhere is the split in Kafka's psyche seen more clearly than when these views about sex and his body are seen alongside his inordinately idealistic conception of marriage ("To have . . . a wife . . . would mean . . . to have God"); he wanted the *hieros gamos,* the sacred marriage (known in alchemy as the *mysterium coniunctionis,* the "mystical" union of the sexes), with none of the carnal element that is an essential part of it when it happens in the outer world. This is reflected in an attitude towards women that was decidedly romantic, and entirely lacking in lust. To Milena he writes, for instance: "I like to hold your hand in mine, I like to look into your eyes. That's about all."[86]

It seems clear from all this that Kafka's ass/greyhound dream compensates a conscious reluctance to accept his earthy, physical, sexual nature. Far from living out this side of himself, he didn't even acknowledge it. Hence the dream is an attempt on the part of the unconscious to redress the imbalance, by drawing his attention to the actual state of affairs; i.e., the over-spiritualization of his dark, chthonic nature. This commonly occurs when one lives too much in the head, and symptomatic bodily disturbances are not the only possible consequences. Psychologically, in the most simple and general terms, Kafka's consciousness was at odds with the unconscious.

Another dream of Kafka's, five years later, shows the two sides at war:

> Two groups of men were fighting each other. The group to which I belonged had captured one of our opponents, a gigantic naked man. Five of us clung to him, one by the head, two on either side by his arms and legs. Unfortunately we had no knife with which to stab him, we hurriedly asked each other for a knife, no one had one. But since for some reason there was no time to lose and an oven stood nearby whose extraordinarily large cast-iron door was red-hot, we dragged the man to it, held one of his feet close to the oven until the foot began to smoke, pulled it back again until it stopped smoking, then thrust it close to the door again. We monotonously kept this up until I awoke, not only in a cold sweat but with my teeth actually chattering. (D2 147-148)

The "two groups of men" represent consciousness and the unconscious, in a state of non-cooperation. The dream ego belongs to consciousness, which has captured "a gigantic naked man." This is reminiscent of Enkidu, the "natural man," the shadow companion Gilgamesh needed to bring him down to earth in order to win his freedom from the mother-goddess Ishtar. Five is associated with the essence of man (head, 2 arms, 2 legs), and this essential humanity, or Anthropos nature, of the giant is emphasized by the positions of those who hold him.

Collectively, in mythological tradition, the Anthropos appears as a cosmic giant, the *prima materia* of the world and the basic substance of all later human generations. The Norse epic *Edda*, for example, describes how the gods shaped the world from the body of the original giant Ymir. In China the dwarf-giant Pan Ku was the cosmic original being: when he wept, the rivers were created; when he breathed, the winds; and when he died, the five sacred mountains emerged from his corpse and his eyes became the sun and the moon. In India the primordial being was the Purusha, and in Persia it was the god-king Gayomart.

Subjectively, the Anthropos is an image of inner divinity; it is connected with nature, the creative essence of the unconscious, and the harmonious interplay of the opposites, especially spirit and matter.[87] It thus represents a primordial psychic unity, a condition of wholeness lost phylogenetically (in the history of mankind) through civilization and the ascent of consciousness, and ontogenetically (in the life of an individual) through growing up. The task of modern man is to rediscover this unity within himself — without the loss of consciousness.

The five men look for a knife with which to stab the giant. The knife is a weapon traditionally used by traitors. It is a phallic symbol, representing aggressive masculinity; also, due to its cutting edge, it is a symbol of discrimination, discernment, and rational thought, as positive aspects of the thinking function. But here its use would obviously be negative, an act of betrayal; in psychological terms it would mean a mental effort to destroy or dismiss the shadow side by intellectual rationalization, theories, and philosophical speculation (thus keeping conflicts in the head). In the dream no knife can be found, indicating a lack of masculinity, and perhaps also suggesting that consciousness does not even recognize the problem. On another level, it may mean that the "sacrifice" of the natural man is not to be permitted.

The five men then resort to a red-hot, cast-iron oven door as an instrument of torture. The oven has numerous associations with the womb and the mother: a pregnant woman is said to have "a bun in her oven"; a woman who has a "fire in her oven" has recently become pregnant; a frigid woman has "a cold oven"; of a woman about to give birth it is said that "her oven is about to cave in"; and an idiot child is said to be "half-baked." Jung writes that "the fiery furnace, like the fiery tripod in *Faust*, is a mother-symbol," the Biblical legend of Shadrach, Meshach, and Abednego in the furnace being "a magical procedure during which a 'fourth' is produced."[88] In the fairytale "The Iron Stove," on the other hand, the oven represents the captive power of the negative feminine (which in that context nevertheless has a positive function, teleologically, in terms of eventual rebirth; what the Church calls a *felix culpa,* a fortunate crime — e.g., Eve eating the apple).

In cooking, the oven is a place where edible food is prepared, a fusion of raw materials. In alchemy the oven is equivalent to the crucible, the *vas Hermetis* (sealed vessel) where the *prima materia* is transformed. This suggests the positive possibilities in terms of the oven if the giant, as a personification of unconscious contents potentially accessible to consciousness, were put inside it. Here, however, far from any concern with transformation, one of his feet is simply roasted until it smokes. (The monotonous, rhythmic motion of the roasting is a motif familiar in fairytales as the "mechanical nodding" of demonic figures; psychologically it points to an "unredeemed" complex that may manifest in meaningless, masochistic suffering.)

The foot, as the organ nearest to the earth, represents the relation to earthly reality, and often has a generative or phallic significance. It is traditionally the weakest part of sun-gods, kings, and heroes, and is often bitten by a snake (Ra) or hit by an arrow (Achilles), or weak (Harpocrates), or deformed (Hephaistus, Oedipus). Wounding of the feet thus suggests a damaged male standpoint; e.g., a malfunctioning sexuality or a recalcitrant creative drive.

Smoke is fantasies (plans "go up in smoke"), laziness ("My days are consumed like smoke" — Psalms 102:3), and evasion ("smokescreen"). In the Bible it is associated with mental darkness (Revelations 9): smoke rises from the "bottomless pit," blinding man's vision of truth, before the terrible locust-demons emerge to devour the unjust.

The alchemists considered smoke to be both soul and spirit *(anima corporalis/spiritualis)* leaving the body.[89] Psychologically, this corresponds to the conscious disidentification of ego from anima and shadow (making possible a relationship between

the ego and these personified aspects of the unconscious). This
is a necessary step, but if the process stops there it is experienced
simply as "loss of soul," i.e., depression. That is why the alchemists speak of the second stage of the *coniunctio*, in which the task
is to re-unite the soul and spirit with the body.[90] In real life,
this means that for insight to have a transformatory effect (and
Kafka had plenty of insights), it must be acted on, taken up into
life. As Jung notes: "Self-knowledge has certain ethical consequences which are not just impassively recognized but demand
to be carried out in practice."[91]

The smoking of the giant's foot is thus, in broad terms, an attempt to depotentiate the "other side" by exposing the "standpoint" of the chthonic shadow to the powerful heat of the
mother-complex. In the earlier dream, the mother principle was
positive, offering life to the ass/greyhound; here it is decidedly
negative, with the five men representing aspects of consciousness
"in the service of the mother." As in the first dream the chthonic
nature represented by the ass was contaminated by the spirit
symbolized by the greyhound, here again the intention seems to
be a spiritualization of the instinct (foot into smoke).

Indeed, so much energy (in the form of heat) is at work in the
unconscious against the shadow, that hardly any libido is available to consciousness. This is reflected in the lysis, the end of the
dream, when Kafka wakes up, "not only in a cold sweat but
with my teeth actually chattering."

The relevance to Kafka's life of the alchemical amplifications
is clear when we realize that in an undifferentiated (unconscious)
man, anima and shadow are experienced as one; any repression,
or rejection, of the unconscious is therefore reflected in loss of
soul. This is what Kafka experienced, not only as depression but
also the pervasive feeling of not being in life; and it is the psychological reality that lay behind his image of the "secret raven."

The task of becoming conscious involves first of all a recogni-
tion of the shadow side of the personality, and also an acknowl-

edgement of its right to live — instead of ignoring, spiritualizing, or fearing its lust for life. Kafka, on the contrary, constantly fought his own "natural man." His idealistic concern for purity, truth, and perfection would not countenance the realities implicit in being a human animal.

As a man consciously assimilates the "earth" of his shadow, he becomes more substantial, more "a man of consequence," i.e., "weighty." (This process may be reflected in dreams in which a shadow figure is seen to have *lost* weight.) The man who does not consciously accept his own shadow lacks earth; he is psychologically without substance, and even his suffering lacks conviction. As Kafka himself expressed it:

> No matter what my complaint, it is without conviction, even without real suffering; like the anchor of a lost ship, it swings far above the bottom in which it could catch hold. (D2 161)

\*

Because Kafka didn't accept his other side, it turned against him. It manifested in real physical ailments ("Strange that the god of pain was not the chief god of the earliest religions" — D2 217), and in feelings of personal worthlessness. "I am sinful in every nook and cranny of my being," he writes in July, 1916. (D2 161) His faults loomed so overlarge in his own eyes that he described himself as "the man with the too-great shadow." (D2 214)

Kafka's self-denigration was usually connected with feelings of his failure as a writer. "When I say something," he notes in July, 1913, "it immediately and finally loses its importance; when I write it down it loses it too." (D1 289) Although he referred to his writing as "a form of prayer" (D1 186) and "my struggle for self-preservation," (D2 75) only on rare occasions did he concede the "saving comfort" of his vocation, and even then in very ambiguous terms:

> The strange, mysterious, perhaps dangerous, perhaps saving
> comfort that there is in writing; it is a leap out of murderer's
> row; it is a seeing of what is really taking place. This occurs by
> a higher type of observation, not a keener type . . . . (D2 212)

More often his writing, and he himself, seemed of little significance; for instance in November, 1913:

> I will write again, but how many doubts have I meanwhile
> had about my writing. At bottom I am an incapable, ignorant
> person who if he had not been compelled — without any ef-
> fort on his own part and scarcely aware of the compulsion —
> to go to school, would be fit only to crouch in a kennel, to
> leap out when food is offered him and to leap back when
> he has swallowed it. (D1 308)

More pointedly in February, 1915:

> At a certain point in self-knowledge, when other circum-
> stances favoring self-scrutiny are present, it will invariably
> follow that you find yourself execrable . . . . You will see
> that you are a rat's nest of miserable dissimulations . . . .
> This filth is the nethermost depth you will find . . . . (D2 114)

And again in September, 1917: "If you insist on digging deep
into yourself, you won't be able to avoid the muck that will
well up." (D2 182)

These self-accusations reveal a sense of inferiority in Kafka,
and are in general symptomatic of *negative inflation.* The term
inflation is commonly used to describe people who have an un-
realistically high opinion of themselves. The extreme cases are
those who believe they are the incarnation of Christ or some
other messiah figure, or have direct telephonic communication
with God. Negative inflation describes the other extreme, that is
identification with one's worst characteristics, one's dark and
shadowy side. It is a typical characteristic of the *puer* with high
ideals that he fails to live up to; the non-acceptance of one's
humanness easily leads to an obsession with one's failings. In the

"dance of life" Kafka drawing reproduced here, for instance, the
male figure is entirely black except for the head — a concrete

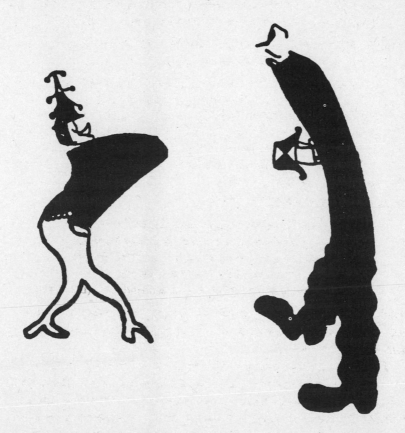

illustration of the "black-and-white" split in Kafka and his attitude towards the body. Note too the man's phallic shape. "Where
there is an undervaluation of sexuality," writes Jung, "the self is
symbolized as a phallus" (e.g., in dreams and drawings):

> Undervaluation can consist in an ordinary repression or in
> overt devaluation . . . . a purely biological interpretation and

evaluation of sexuality can also have this effect. Any such conception overlooks the spiritual and "mystical" implications of the sexual instinct.[92]

Kafka's view of sex, as we have seen, was strictly biological, hence his remark about "coitus as punishment . . . . "
    Regarding inflation, Jung has the following comments:

> An inflated consciousness is always egocentric and conscious of nothing but its own existence. It is incapable of learning from the past, incapable of understanding contemporary events, and incapable of drawing right conclusions about the future. It is hypnotized by itself and therefore cannot be argued with. It inevitably dooms itself to calamities that must strike it dead.
>
> Paradoxically enough, inflation is a regression of consciousness into unconsciousness. This always happens when consciousness takes too many unconscious contents upon itself and loses the faculty of discrimination, the *sine qua non* of all consciousness.[93]

Inflation of either kind is therefore a form of possession, and indicates an urgent need to consciously assimilate unconscious shadow characteristics.

Assimilation is the reverse of identification; it involves becoming objective about one's complexes instead of being possessed by them. This leads to a change of attitude towards oneself, and like any change of attitude it cannot be done in the head; it must be an experiential, feeling realization. Writes Jung:

> Feeling always binds one to the reality and meaning of symbolic contents, and these in turn impose binding standards of ethical behaviour from which aestheticism and intellectualism are only too ready to emancipate themselves.[94]

That is why the analytical process, for instance, when pursued on an intellectual level — and that includes most self-analysis — is inevitably sterile:

> As long as an analysis moves on the mental plane nothing
> happens, you can discuss whatever you please, it makes no
> difference, but when you strike against something below the
> surface, then a thought comes up in the form of an experience,
> and stands before you like an object . . . . Whenever you ex-
> perience a thing that way, you know instantly that it is a
> fact.[95]

Such "thoughts in the form of an experience" have a trans-
forming effect because they are numinous, that is overwhelm-
ing. They lead to a more balanced perspective: one is merely
human — not entirely good (positive inflation), not entirely bad
(negative inflation), but a homogenous amalgam of good and
evil. The realization and acceptance of this is a mark of the inte-
grated personality.

In Kafka, who placed so much emphasis on perfection rather
than integration (or wholeness), the effect was to constellate
what may be seen as "the dark side of God," which constantly
threatened to overwhelm him — in order, compensatorily, to
bring him down to earth. The struggle Kafka waged within himself was the result of an intransigent conscious attitude. Under
these conditions, with virtually no degree of conscious understanding and assimilation of what was happening to him, his
search for life was, as he himself describes it, a torturing,
Tantalus situation:

> He is thirsty, and is cut off from a spring by a mere clump
> of bushes. But he is divided against himself: one part over-
> looks the whole, sees that he is standing here and that the
> spring is just beside him; but another part notices nothing,
> has at most a divination that the first part sees all. But as he
> notices nothing he cannot drink.[96]

The spring, of course, contains the water of life. Water itself is a
widespread symbol for the unconscious, the source of renewal.
Kafka, "divided against himself," is cut off from the healing
waters by "a mere clump of bushes" — bushes, like trees in gen-

eral, having a maternal significance, and here relating to the confining effect of the mother-complex.

And yet, Kafka held out. Some inner force continued to sustain him. He called it "hope":

> Insoluble problem: Am I broken? Am I in decline? Almost
> all the signs speak for it (coldness, apathy, state of my nerves,
> distractedness, incompetence on the job, headaches, insomnia);
> almost nothing but hope speaks against it. (D2 140)

Or alternatively, in one of his "Reflections on Sin, Pain, Hope, and the True Way":

> Man cannot live without an enduring trust in something indestructible in himself. Yet while doing that he may all his life
> be unaware of that indestructible thing and of his trust in it.[97]

That "something indestructible" is, in psychological terms, what Jung called the Self.

# 3 THE PROVISIONAL LIFE AND THE FEMININE

While on holiday in Denmark in July, 1914, Kafka drafted to his parents (but never sent) a revealing letter in which he envisioned a bold plan: to leave Prague for Berlin, marry Felice Bauer, and manage as best they could on the money he'd saved, selling his work if possible. This letter is important not only because it shows that Kafka did not entirely dismiss the possibility of earning a living by his literary work, but because it also shows a clear awareness of what was at stake in his life:

> So far I have grown up in complete dependence and outward well-being . . . . The only good [!] result of dependence is that it keeps one young . . . . Here everything is arranged to keep me, a man that fundamentally asks for dependence, in that state. Everything is so nicely laid to my hand. The office I find very burdensome and often unbearable, but at bottom, all the same, easy. In this way I earn more than I need. What for? Whom for? I shall go up in the scale of salaries. To what purpose?
>
> If this work doesn't suit me and doesn't even bring independence as a reward, why should I not throw it up? I have nothing to risk, and everything to gain if I hand in my resignation and go away from Prague. I risk nothing because my life in Prague leads to nothing good.[98]

Quite true, perhaps — but the plan fell through with the outbreak of war, and there is no reason to believe Kafka could, or would, have carried it out anyway. For even if he had had the physical strength necessary to act on his insight, and even if he hadn't been ambivalent about the girl, one doubts that he had a genuine desire to change what he recognized (here and elsewhere) as his situation of "complete dependence."

## THE PRISON

"Dependence" was for Kafka equivalent to imprisonment. In October, 1916, he writes to Felice Bauer: "I, who for the most part have been a dependent creature, have an infinite yearning for independence and freedom in all things." (D2 166-167) Max Brod feels that this conflict (security/freedom) could have been resolved "had he been allowed to let his artistic capabilities have their full run,"[99] but in fact the dichotomy lies at the very heart of his neurosis, and the image of a prison is a key one in understanding it.

I have already quoted Kafka's lament that "an unfortunate man, one who is condemned to have no children, is terribly imprisoned in his own misfortune." Recall too the conversation with Gustav Janouch in which Kafka describes his parental home as "a prison specially constructed for myself," and observes that "one cannot break one's chains when there are no chains to be seen." Such "chains," of course, are actually unconscious ties to the parents and the security they represent — ties that must be severed in order to grow up and lead an independent life. Hence the experience of life as imprisonment is a ubiquitous motif in the psychology of the *puer aeternus*.

About the same time as that conversation with Janouch (1920), Kafka wrote the following aphorism:

> He could have resigned himself to a prison. To end as a prisoner — that could be a life's ambition. But it was a barred cage that he was in. Calmly and insolently, as if at home, the din of the world streamed out and in through the bars, the prisoner was really free, he could take in everything, nothing that went on outside escaped him, he could simply have left the cage, the bars were yards apart, he was not even a prisoner.[100]

This passage, typical of Kafka's mind-twisting, paradoxical style, is a significant picture of "negative" imprisonment, suggesting a man trapped, locked up in his own psyche, with only himself as his keeper. He is really free to come and go as he pleases, but he doesn't make a move.

By way of contrast, look at this verse from Lovelace's poem, "To Althea from Prison":

> Stone Walls do not a Prison make,
> Nor Iron bars a Cage,
> Mindes innocent and quiet take
> That for an Hermitage.
> If I have freedome in my Love,
> And in my soul am free,
> Angels alone that sore above
> Injoy such Liberty.[101]

These lines speak of a sense of freedom in spite of being behind bars. Kafka's image mourns a loss of freedom in spite of *not* being behind bars. Another of Kafka's aphorisms, from the feeling side, is less enigmatic:

> He feels imprisoned on this earth, he feels constricted; the
> melancholy, the impotence, the sicknesses, the feverish fan-
> cies of the captive afflict him; no comfort can comfort him,
> since it is merely comfort, gentle head-splitting comfort
> glossing the brutal fact of imprisonment. But if he is asked
> what he actually wants he cannot reply, for — that is one of
> his strongest proofs — he has no conception of freedom.[102]

The prison is a symbol familiar enough to the analyst. Jung refers to it as one among the many possible quaternary images of the Self,[103] but this is true only as long as fear of the Self still prevails. In other words, a sense of imprisonment indicates a *refusal* of the individuation process. This refusal is in fact symptomatic of the psychology of the *puer;* behind it is a disinclination to grow up and assume personal responsibility for oneself. Kafka, for instance, while acknowledging in the *Letter to His Father* that "marriage certainly is the pledge of the most acute form of self-liberation and independence,"[104] claimed that marrying was barred to him simply because it was his father's domain:

> Sometimes I imagine the map of the world spread out and you
> stretched diagonally across it. And I feel as if I could consider
> living in only those regions that either are not covered by you
> or are not within your reach.[105]

To marry, he observed, would make him his father's equal, but
that "would be like a fairytale . . . . It is too much; so much cannot be achieved" — and again he uses the image of imprisonment:

> It is as if a person were a prisoner, and he had not only the
> intention to escape, which would perhaps be attainable, but
> also, and indeed simultaneously, the intention to rebuild the
> prison as a pleasure dome for himself. But if he escapes, he
> cannot rebuild, and if he rebuilds, he cannot escape.[106]

With regard to his engagement to Felice Bauer, on the other
hand, the list cited earlier — reasons "for and against" his marriage — makes it clear that the "just-so story" of earthly reality was completely unacceptable to him, for his sense of freedom
was intimately connected with lack of limitations. As he notes
in his diary in January, 1915:

> I yield not a particle of my demand for a fantastic life ar-
> ranged solely in the interest of my work; she, indifferent to
> every mute request, wants the average: a comfortable home,
> an interest on my part in the factory, good food, bed at
> eleven, central heating; sets my watch — which for the past
> three months has been an hour and a half fast — right to the
> minute. And she is right in the end and would continue to be
> right in the end. (D2 111-112)

The implication here is that an on-going relationship would involve intolerable restrictions. But looked at from a psychological point of view, such "restrictions" are the very param-
eters of growth. In the language of the *I Ching* (Hexagram 60,
Limitation):

Unlimited possibilities are not suited to man; if they existed,
his life would only dissolve in the boundless. To become strong,
a man's life needs the limitations ordained by duty and voluntarily accepted. The individual attains significance as a free
spirit only by surrounding himself with these limitations and
by determining for himself what his duty is.[107]

In these terms, Kafka's "prison" was neither his job nor his
parental home nor his childless fate. It was an attitude of mind —
an adolescent attitude that refused to accept any limits, therefore chafed at any limitation at all. This is the other face of
Kafka's stiff ego stance that refused to take the unconscious seriously. They both come to the same thing: hybris, symptomatic of an
inflated ego.

Adrift on a sea of boundless possibilities, Kafka was beset by
the agonies of frustration. Recall the diary entry: "Impossible to
live with F. Intolerable living with anyone. I don't regret this; I
regret the impossibility for me of not living alone." (D2 157)
Neither a prisoner nor yet in life, Kafka suffered what he described as "not death, alas, but the endless torment of dying." (D2 77)

Marie Louise von Franz maintains that for the man who remains too long in adolescent psychology it cannot be any other
way. She describes the prison phobia of a young mother-bound
man, and remarks:

The prison is the negative symbol of the mother-complex . . .
or it would be prospectively just exactly what he needs, for
he needs to be put into prison, into the prison of reality.
But if he runs away from the prison of reality, he is in the
prison of his mother-complex, so it is prison anyway, where-
ever he turns. He has only the choice of two prisons, either
that of his neurosis or that of his reality; thus he is caught
between the devil and the deep blue sea. That is his fate, and
that is the fate of the *puer aeternus* altogether. It is up to him
which he prefers: that of his mother-complex and his neurosis,
or of being caught in the just-so story of earthly reality.[108]

There is a difference, however. In the prison of the mother-complex there is only masochistic suffering, while in the prison of earthly reality there is the possibility of transformation — after which reality and its limitations are no longer experienced as imprisonment.

Indeed, it is precisely through limitation, according to the *I Ching* passage quoted above, that a man "attains significance as a free spirit." In metaphorical terms, this means he finds "the treasure" — the inner gold, the Self.

In some early seminars on basic psychological principles, Jung relates the concept of the lost treasure to projection, loss of soul, and the fear of imprisonment:

> When you are in the condition of the beginning of life, in an adolescent condition of mind, you are not in possession of the animus — or the anima in a man's case — and you have no consciousness of the Self, because they are both projected. You are then . . . liable to become possessed by somebody who seems to contain these values; you get under the influence of the apparent proprietors of your treasures, and that is of course a sort of magic influence.
>
> Now the more you get under that fascination, the more you become immovable . . . . You are in prison, you are utterly unfree.
>
> That is why people are afraid of each other — they fear that somebody could put them into prison. Many people have a tremendous fear of attaching themselves, they fear the loss not only of their mental freedom, but of their moral and spiritual freedom, as if the very soul were threatened . . . .
>
> But if you can accept the fact of being caught, of course you are imprisoned, but on the other hand you have a chance to come into possession of your treasures. There is no other way; you never will come into possession of your treasures if you keep aloof, if you run about like a wild dog.[109]

This would explain the *puer*'s characteristic fear of being grounded — i.e., imprisoned or trapped — by a relationship with a woman. In just such terms did Kafka express his feelings about the opposite sex:

> Women are snares, which lie in wait for men on all sides in order to drag them into the merely finite. They lose their dangers if one voluntarily falls into one of the snares. But if, as a result of habit, one overcomes it, then all the jaws of the female trap open again.[110]

The "merely finite" is a wonderful expression for the limitations felt by a man when he commits himself to a woman. In fantasy, unattached, the possibilities are infinite. Anything less is experienced as a sacrifice, a more or less intolerable loss of freedom. According to an old alchemical saying, "The male is the heaven [spirit] of the female, and the female is the earth of the male."[111] This means that the connection with a woman has the effect of bringing a man down to earth. The man who is psychologically reluctant to be grounded, as is the *puer,* lives in a kind of limbo that only the right woman can rescue him from — and the "right" woman is seldom the one he has in mind. Meanwhile he suffers the torment of the damned, for the inability to sustain a true connection does not still the yearning.

In the passage quoted above, what Kafka calls the "jaws of the female trap" is analogous to the dreaded *vagina dentata,* a vagina with teeth, a ubiquitous symbol corresponding psychologically to the devouring mother, and in this context directly relevant to Kafka's sexual problem. As von Franz notes:

> In the male, sex with aggression can be combined, but not sex and fear. In the female, sex and fear can be combined, but not aggression and sex. And there you have the animus-anima problem in a nutshell.[112]

We know that Kafka was not at all aggressive, a consequence of the lack of contact with his chthonic shadow. And we also know that the rejection of his animal nature was reflected in his more or less obsessive concern with "perfection." The overall result was a severe inhibition of the instincts that must certainly have contributed substantially to his sense of imprisonment. For his body, in a very real sense, was locked up.

Jung, describing the peculiar feeling of "being caught" that often accompanies the process of coming to terms with the reality of oneself, stresses the importance of accepting bodily limitations:

> When people come to themselves they expect a peculiar liberation, to be free from responsibilities, and from vices and virtues, but in reality it is quite different. It is like a trap, you suddenly fall into a hole. "Hang it all!" you say, and there you are, where you belong . . . . The hole which one falls into is through the body, and the body says "but this *is* you." All this is expressed by the prison.[113]

Without the body, the spirit lacks substance; without spirit, the body is an empty vessel. A conscious involvement with both — and dealing with the inevitable conflicts — is a mark of the individuating personality.

Kafka did finally come down to earth. He found and loved a woman; he "voluntarily" grounded himself — or fell into one of the snares. In the process, by all accounts, he also experienced a sense of freedom that belied his earlier fears and gave him a new lease on life. His prison bars vanished, as it were; he found some of his treasures.

Until then, he suffered, but he never gave up hope. As expressed in a diary entry in 1920:

> It is no disproof of one's presentiment of an ultimate liberation
> if the next day one's imprisonment continues on unchanged,
> or is even made straiter, or if it is even expressly stated that
> it will never end. All this can rather be the necessary preliminary to an ultimate liberation. (D2 193)

Nor indeed was this an ill-founded expectation, mythologically speaking. Sun-gods and heroes, too, commonly suffered a period of imprisonment — or Descent into Hell — before "ultimate liberation." It is a well-known variation of the "night sea journey" motif,[114] and Osiris, Christ, Jonah, Dante, Odysseus, Aeneas, and countless others are all in the same boat, so to speak, as anyone who endures a severe depression.

All the night sea journey myths derive ultimately from the perceived behaviour of the sun, which, in Jung's lyrical image, "sails over the sea like an immortal god who every evening is immersed in the maternal waters and is born anew in the morning."[115]

The sun going down, seen psychologically as the loss of energy accompanying depression, is thus a necessary prelude to rebirth. The mere mortal, however, as distinct from the sun, is never all that sure he will rise again.


## THE PROVISIONAL LIFE

The *puer*'s fear of being grounded usually goes hand in hand with a stubborn and fearful reluctance to stand on his own two feet. It is an attitude of mind not unlike that found among institutionalized patients who become so accustomed to being taken care of that they aren't able to leave. In Kafka's case, it kept him living at home and dependent on his parents (or at times his youngest sister Ottilie), and tied to a job that involved what he described as "a horrible double life from which there is probably no escape but insanity." (D1 44)

Kafka did not go insane, but he was certainly suffering neurotically, for he was caught in what Jung called "the provisional life": one's lot is not what one really wants; one is always "about to" take the step into real life; some day one will do what is necessary — only not just yet. Plans for the future never reach fruition, life slips away in endless fantasies of what will be, what could be, while no decisive action is ever taken to change the present.

Some people go on like this forever, with no trouble at all. For the most part, however, the provisional life simply does not work; the unconscious eventually rebels and makes its dissatisfaction apparent through physical or emotional symptoms. As Jung writes in *The Visions Seminars:*

> The immediate things are this earth, this life. For quite long enough our ancestors — and we ourselves — have been taught that this life is not the real thing, that it is provisional, and that we only live for heaven. It is because our whole [Christian] morality has been based on that negation of the flesh that our unconscious so often works to convince us of the importance of living here and now. For, in the course of the centuries, man has repeatedly experienced that the life which is not lived here, the life which is lived as something provisional, is utterly unsatisfactory, that it leads to neurosis . . . . As long as it is a case of provisional life your unconscious will be in a state of continuous irritation.[116]

Von Franz points out that in a person living the provisional life there is always a "but" that prevents marriage or any kind of definite commitment:

> There is always the fear of being caught in a situation from which it may be impossible to slip out again. Every just-so situation is hell. . . . For the time being one is doing this or that, but whether it is a woman or a job, it is *not yet* what is really wanted, and there is always the fantasy that sometime in the future the real thing will come about.[117]

If this attitude is prolonged it means a constant inner refusal to commit oneself to the moment. Under such conditions there is no sense of being in life; it is as if one were not yet born.

Kafka had exactly that feeling. In January, 1922, he writes in his diary: "Hesitation before birth. If there is a transmigration of souls then I am not yet on the bottom rung. My life is a hesitation before birth." (D2 210) Again, in February, 1922: "In the Great Account of my life, it is still reckoned as if my life were

first beginning tomorrow." (D2 222) And a month later, most
pointedly: "Still unborn and already compelled to walk around
the streets and speak to people." (D2 225)

H.G. Baynes, one of Jung's earliest students, a medical doctor
and author of the monumental *Mythology of the Soul*, has pre-
sented a case study of a patient living the provisional life. Here
he writes that such people are inclined to complain that

> the circumstances of their life, their ill-health, their intense
> sympathy for the suffering of others, their extreme sensitivity
> to noise, light, heat, cold, psychic atmosphere, climate, con-
> stipation, insomnia and the rest, all conspire to prevent them
> from living a normal responsible existence.[118]

— in accordance with which, a sizable dossier could be compiled
on Kafka, beginning with his hypochondria, as already noted.
Kafka's "sensitivity to noise" was in fact particularly acute, as
witness this early diary entry:

> I want to write, with a constant trembling on my forehead.
> I sit in my room in the very headquarters of the uproar of the
> entire house. I hear all the doors close, because of their noise
> only the footsteps of those running between them are spared
> me, I hear even the slamming of the oven door in the kitchen.
> My father bursts through the doors of my room and passes
> through in his dragging dressing gown, the ashes are scraped
> out of the stove in the next room, Valli asks, shouting into the
> indefinite through the anteroom as though through a Paris
> street, whether father's hat has been brushed yet, a hushing
> that claims to be friendly to me raises the shout of an answer-
> ing voice. The house door is unlatched and screeches as though
> from a catarrhal throat, then opens wider with the brief sing-
> ing of a woman's voice and closes with a dull manly jerk that
> sounds most inconsiderate. My father is gone, now begins the
> more delicate, more distracted, more hopeless noise led by
> the voices of the two canaries. I had already thought of it
> before, but with the canaries it comes back to me again, that

> I might open the door a narrow crack, crawl into the next
> room like a snake and in that way, on the floor, beg my
> sisters and their governess for quiet. (D1 133)

This passage is hyperbolic, to be sure, and redolent of Kafka's
gift for comic irony, but nonetheless an illustration of how Kafka
experienced his situation; namely, as a man being pummelled by
deafening distractions.

Baynes also notes:

> To live provisionally means to depute to the unconscious
> just those functions of realization and responsibility that
> are needed for navigating an intelligent and effective course.
> The place which these functions should occupy in conscious-
> ness is filled, instead, by fuss and self-justification.[119]

The particular "functions of realization and responsibility"
that are "deputed" to the unconscious (i.e., lost to the ego) will
of course depend on the typology of the individual concerned.
Kafka was almost certainly an introverted intuitive (von Franz:
"the type of the religious prophet"[120]), and as such his inferior
function was extraverted sensation, the *fonction du réel*. This
means he was bound to have difficulty in accepting his existen-
tial reality — the here and now — and it may even have contributed to his tuberculosis. As noted by one analyst in a study of
the clinical significance of introversion and extraversion:

> It is perhaps possible that the introvert — in order to remain
> calm and aloof from the world — breathes in an inadequate
> and inhibited way, and thus may become relatively easily
> susceptible to pulmonary tuberculosis.[121]

It must be mentioned here too that although the infection in
Kafka's lungs was a cold, hard fact, like any physical symptom it
may be viewed symbolically. We know that Kafka's "spiritual"
search, through his writing, was virtually his only concern. We
know too that his conscious attitude was impoverished by the
non-acceptance of his shadow side. The lungs (*phrenes*), as the

seat of the *pneuma* (breath, spirit), were considered by the early
Greeks to be the centre of not only thinking and emotion but
also of consciousness (the "blood-soul") in general.[122] With this
in mind, contamination of the lungs would indicate a condition
of disharmony between body and spirit.

Kafka himself was not blind to the symbolic significance of
his illness, though he expressed it rather more concretely:

> If the infection in your lungs is only a symbol, as you say, a
> symbol of the infection whose inflammation is called F. and
> whose depth is its deep justification; if this is so then the medi-
> cal advice (light, air, sun, rest) is also a symbol. Lay hold of
> this symbol. (D2 182)

But whatever the symbolism involved in Kafka's tuberculosis,
it is clear that for the most part he did not accept the reality
of his life; and acceptance of what exists is the necessary prelude
to change. Hence Kafka remained in a psychological impasse, ex-
emplified by what he called "complete dependence," a man
constantly at odds with himself.

In many ways this is puzzling, for one could not say that Kafka
was *unaware* of his reality; on the contrary, he described it in no
uncertain terms. He also had a good idea of what to do about it.
"Rise up, then," he writes in his diary in August, 1916. "Mend
your ways, escape officialdom, start seeing what you are instead
of calculating what you should become." (D2 164) And Gustav
Janouch quotes Kafka as saying: "Reality is never and nowhere
more accessible than in the immediate moment of one's own
life" [123] — a profound observation that made hardly a dent in
his own "provisionality" at the time (1921).

"It is almost as if, for most people, the discovery of reality
were a cause for panic," writes Jung:

> The interesting thing is that if you tell such a thing to people
> who are living the provisional life, they nod their heads wisely
> and know all about it; then they go right on as they were, they
> continue their sleep.[124]

To fall asleep corresponds psychologically to becoming unconscious. Was Kafka, then, "asleep," in this sense, for most of his
life? If so, it may account for the form, and often the content, of
his writing. (Interestingly enough, at one point Kafka expressed
a desire to write his autobiography, "because it would move along
as easily as the writing down of dreams." (D1 181)

"To admit reality into one's life," observes Baynes, "means to
take responsibility for something and to serve it unconditionally":

> And this means to be shaped and, perhaps, even transformed
> by an unknown power. This is the very core of the neurotic
> fear of life, the dread lest something should so seize hold of
> the mind that one might be carried away and delivered over
> irrevocably to an unknown and unpredictable fate. At bot-
> tom, *it is the ego's yearning dread of the Self.*[125]

— and with that we are back to the prison as a negative image
of the Self, indicating a refusal to become what one potentially
is; i.e., fear of the process of individuation.

With this fear, indeed, may be connected what Kafka called,
in the *Letter to His Father*, his "boundless sense of guilt."[126]
Kafka himself laid the blame for this at his father's door — a
typical *puer* evasion of responsibility. But the psychological
reality is that individuation demands the living out of one's potential on both fronts, the inner and the outer, and Kafka committed himself to neither. Thus he suffered a sense of guilt from
not being a more "productive" member of society, and also because he allowed outside activities to distract him from exploit-
ing his literary talent to the full.

The more one throws oneself into life, the more one is liable
to make mistakes, to do things wrong. That is the unavoidable
consequence of being "in life." By not living, by hiding behind
bars, Kafka did not accumulate much *active* guilt, rather he was
the victim of *passive* guilt. His novel *The Trial*, for instance, develops this feeling with consummate skill: What K., the "hero,"
has done is never said, never discovered. By ordinary civil stan-

dards he is undoubtedly innocent, yet he *feels* guilty and makes every effort to atone for he-knows-not-what. As Kafka wrote of himself when he broke off his first engagement to Felice Bauer: "There was nothing, or not much, that could be said against me. Devilish in my innocence." (D2 65)

Von Franz, in making this distinction between active and passive guilt, writes of the *puer*: "He has not done all those things that a more virile man might perhaps have done, but . . . . he has committed the sin of not living." [127] Similarly, Kafka's pervasive sense of guilt may be seen as a consequence of his "unlived life."

Anything may be viewed psychologically from two points of view, causal and prospective. Whatever the cause of Kafka's guilt feelings, their prospective function would be to prod him into taking action; i.e., rearrange the real circumstances of his life so that it was, for him, more meaningful. But Kafka did not leave the prison of his provisional life until he was nearly dead. In fact, one might say he wallowed in it — and paid accordingly.

"The criterion of adulthood," writes Jung, "does not consist in being a member of certain sects, groups, or nations, but in submitting to the spirit of one's own independence." [128] Kafka had that spirit, he acknowledged it, but until it was almost too late he was unable to do anything about it.

"Every man lives behind bars, which he carries within him," said Kafka to Janouch (commenting on David Garnett's story, *Lady into Fox*). "That is why people write so much about animals now." (As Kafka did himself — e.g., his *Investigations of a Dog; Report to an Academy* (an ape); *The Metamorphosis* (a cockroach); *The Giant Mole; Josephine the Singer* (a mouse); and *The Burrow* (another mole); to mention only the longer stories.) Kafka continued:

> It's an expression of longing for a free natural life . . . . Human existence is a burden to them, so they dispose of it in fantasies . . . . Men are afraid of freedom and responsibility. So they

prefer to hide behind the prison bars which they build around themselves.[129]

And there can be little doubt that here he was speaking of himself.

Kafka, a man with "an infinite yearning for independence and freedom," was yet afraid of freedom and evaded the responsibility inherent in his creative gift. That is the paradox Kafka lived out — as he counselled himself not to give up:

> If you were walking over a plain with the honest desire to make progress, and yet found yourself further back than when you started, then it would be a hopeless business; but as you are clambering up a steep precipice, as steep, say, as you yourself seen from below, your backward slips may only be caused after all by the lie of the land, and you must not despair.[130]

## THE MOTHER AND THE ANIMA

Behind Kafka's provisional life, behind his dependence and the fear of individuation, lay the mother-complex. Its effect was to cut him off from life. It was as if there were a plastic envelope between him and reality so that he was never quite in touch with the real world, and never wholly committed to anything. As we have seen, Kafka experienced this as a form of imprisonment.

Indeed, the effect of any complex is to limit freedom. To the extent that one is conscious of one's own psychology, one is able to function with a degree of self-determination. To the extent that one is manipulated by unconscious forces (complexes), one is in bondage, there is no freedom at all.

According to Jung, the mother-complex manifests most typically in Don Juanism, homosexuality, and sometimes also impotence. But a man with a strong mother-complex may have a finely differentiated Eros instead of, or in addition to, homosexuality. This can give him a great capacity for friendship, which often, writes Jung, "creates astonishing tenderness between men and may even rescue friendship between the sexes from the limbo of the impossible."[131] The mother-complex may also endow a man with "a wealth of religious feelings . . . and a spiritual receptivity which makes him responsive to revelation."[132]

Similarly, what appears negatively as Don Juanism can manifest positively as ambitious striving after the highest goals (the "truth"); a willingness to make sacrifices for what is regarded as right (heroism); perseverance, inflexibility, and toughness of will; a healthy curiosity; and finally, writes Jung, "a revolutionary spirit which strives to put a new face upon the world."[133]

In Kafka's case, there is the possibility of impotence, but no question of Don Juanism. There are some indications in his life and diaries of a homosexual orientation — particularly in the close friendship with Max Brod — but no evidence at all of overt homosexuality. As one study notes:

> He may very well have had latent homosexual impulses that occasionally expressed themselves in displaced or symbolic ways, but this would not distinguish Kafka from the bulk of mankind.[134]

He was, however, as Max Brod and others testify, capable of "astonishing tenderness" towards his male friends.[135]

The positive effects of Kafka's mother-complex are immediately apparent in his high ideals (both personal and collective), and what may be described in broad terms as "religious strivings." This is generally true of the *puer*, and not surprisingly, for his connection with the mother principle gives him a close contact with the unconscious and the springs of creativity; so he is often a sensitive searcher for spirit.

For Kafka, this search and his writing were virtually inseparable. "Writing as a form of prayer," he notes in his diary. (D1 186) One critic describes the essence of his work as "truthfulness: the

striving for truth and nothing else."[136] Max Brod refers to
Kafka's religion, "in the sense of a properly fulfilled life," as his
"decisive message."[137] Art for Kafka, attests Brod, was "a way
to God"[138]; behind Kafka's "literary mandate," writes Brod,
lies a religious question —

> a religious question after the peculiar quality of Kafka's re-
> ligion, which was a religion of the life fulfilled, of work,
> good work, that fulfils life significantly, of co-ordination
> in the right and proper life of national and human communi-
> ty.[139]

And this type of life is precisely what Kafka did not experience.
Hence his longing for children ("Nowhere a hope for revival, for
help from luckier stars . . . .") may be seen as a form of compensation for his own unlived life, and therefore symbolic of his
need for psychic rebirth.

Rebirth means new life, and for a man this happens through
the process of differentiating his moods and emotions in order
to know what he really wants. This can take him out of his "prison" and reveal the unreality of the "provisional life."

But this requires energy, libido. And as long as the libido is
tied up by the mother-complex, as it was in Kafka's case, it is
not consciously available for other purposes. Kafka's image, already noted, of "the dirty unknown old woman with shrunken
thighs who drains his semen in an instant," and "pockets the
money," is in fact a remarkably suitable metaphor for the drain
of energy by the mother-complex.

In the world of ideas, the realm of religious speculation and
anguish, Kafka was independent. But psychologically he was not
his own man because he was under the thumb of the mother-
complex. That is why, in spite of the lack of affinity with his
parents, he experienced the greatest difficulty in living away
from home. For there, in his self-styled prison, he was effectively protected from the necessity of having to grapple with, and

mould to his own bidding, the male-oriented, outside world.  As
Jung writes in *Aion:*

> [The real world] makes demands on the masculinity of a man,
> on his ardour, above all on his courage and resolution when
> it comes to throwing his whole being into the scales. For this
> he would need a faithless Eros, one capable of forgetting his
> mother and undergoing the pain of relinquishing the first love
> of his life.[140]

\*

In a lecture delivered in 1936, Jung states that from the psychological point of view there are five main groups of instinctive
factors: hunger, sexuality, activity, reflection, and creativity. The
creative instinct, writes Jung, is, like the other instincts, "com-
pulsive, but it is not common, and it is not a fixed and invariably
inherited organization":

> It has much in common with the drive to activity and the
> reflective instinct. But it can also suppress them, or make
> them serve it to the point of the self-destruction of the in-
> dividual. Creation is as much destruction as construction.[141]

Certainly, Kafka felt this to be true. Writing — his "artificial,
miserable substitute . . . for forebears, marriage and heirs" — was
a compulsion with him, and apparently not inherited. And although he had to have long periods of time in order to write, he
realized that a preoccupation with himself and "literature"
thwarted his personal development in other ways.

It is not with pride, for instance, that Kafka notes in December, 1911: "I look at my whole way of life going in a direction
that is foreign and false to all my relatives and acquaintances."
(D1 185) He profoundly regretted the extent to which he neglected other aspects of life. "Who is to confirm for me the truth
or probability of this," he writes in March, 1912, "that it is only
because of my literary mission that I am uninterested in all things,
and therefore heartless?" (D1 245) And in August, 1914:

> My talent for portraying my dreamlike inner life has thrust
> all other matters into the background; my life has dwindled
> dreadfully, nor will it cease to dwindle. (D2 77)

But he adds, all the same: "Nothing else will ever satisfy me."

Here is the heart of Kafka's "two worlds" conflict. His basic dilemma — the tragedy of his life, one might say — was that he admired and wanted a life of peaceable simplicity (or "normality"), while he was tormented by a nature that sought something else, demanded something more. And he could not reconcile the two. "I am still going in two directions," he notes in November, 1917. "The work awaiting me is enormous." (D2 190) "There is a goal," runs one of his aphorisms, "but no way; what we call the way is only wavering."[142] Another:

> The true way goes over a rope which is not stretched at any
> great height but just above the ground. It seems more design-
> ed to make people stumble than to be walked upon.[143]

(By way of contrast, compare Jung's view: "The goal is important only as an idea; the essential thing is the *opus* [i.e., the work on oneself] which leads to the goal: *that* is the goal of a lifetime."[144])

In *The Wisdom of the Heart*, Henry Miller writes:

> Art is only a means to life, to the life more abundant. It is
> not in itself the life more abundant. It merely points the
> way, something which is overlooked not only by the public,
> but very often by the artist himself.[145]

Far from overlooking this, Kafka could not forget it, for he did not believe (as for instance Rilke did) in the primacy of art, "art for art's sake." Writing was the vocation to which Kafka was irresistably drawn, it was the focal point of his life — but to him it was not life in any real, satisfactory sense, and by no means "the life more abundant."

Psychologically, the function that takes a man into life is the anima, his soul. Jung describes the anima as "the archetype of life itself."[146] A person full of life is "animated"; to be without the anima is experienced as lifelessness ("loss of soul") and depression — Kafka's dominant state.

In his diary in October, 1921, Kafka mourns the empty years and inner turmoil, expressing his never-ending hope for release in terms that invoke his lost soul:

> It is entirely conceivable that life's splendor forever lies in wait about each one of us in all its fulness, but veiled from view, deep down, invisible, far off. It *is* there, though, not hostile, not reluctant, not deaf. If you summon it by the right word, by its right name, it will come. This is the essence of magic, which does not create but su:.imons. (D2 195)

"Life's splendor" is a wonderful image for the anima as a positive life force. She does "lie in wait"; and it is true that she is "not hostile, not reluctant, not deaf." But she demands attention, and until she gets it she remains "veiled from view" — lost to consciousness because of a wrong attitude. The magic word to summon her is simple enough — "Hello" — and once summoned and related to, she can not only take a man into life but also function in her capacity as creative muse.

The more contact a man has with his anima — i.e., the more he differentiates his experience of himself — the more she develops. In terms of this psychological development, Jung has personified four "stages" of the anima: Eve, Helen, Mary, and Sophia.[147]

In the first stage, Eve, the man's anima is wholly contaminated with the mother-imago. This manifests in a man's inability to function independently. In the second, as Helen, she is a collective sexual figure. ("All is dross that is not Helen" — Marlowe). A man with such an anima may exhaust himself with repeated, and short-lived, sexual adventures. In the third stage, as Mary, there is the possibility of personal relationships free of projection. And in the fourth, the anima as Sophia (known to the Gnostics as "Mother of Wisdom") functions as psychopomp (guide), mediating to consciousness the contents of the collective unconscious; in this guise she fulfils her role as the artist's muse.

In theory, a man's anima development proceeds stage by stage, and over a long period this can be seen to be true. In practice, however, a man may have periodic contact with any of these stages — depending, compensatorily, on his particular conscious attitude — and indeed, the concept of wholeness involves experiencing them all.

Kafka aimed high from the start — right at Sophia. That seems clear enough in light of his "soul-searching" and "spiritual strivings," which began at an early age. His single-mindedness in this respect strongly suggests that he was possessed by this aspect of the anima. This happens when a man identifies himself absolutely with his reason and his spirituality, and commonly results in losing touch altogether with the compensating powers of the unconscious. "In such cases," writes Jung,

> the unconscious usually responds with violent emotions, irritability, lack of control, arrogance, feelings of inferiority, moods, depressions, outbursts of rage, etc., coupled with lack of self-criticism and the misjudgments, mistakes, and delusions which this entails.[148]

This condition is aptly characterized as a "suffering of the soul," which if ignored eventually manifests in more serious physical or psychological sympto s that demand immediate attention. Even at this point, however, it is characteristic of the neurotic mind to merely note the suffering, without becoming conscious of the reasons behind it or taking any action. This development is typical of *puer* psychology, of which Kafka is such a classic example. (It can also be observed, notes Jung, "among so-called normal people who have come into conflict with the unconscious thanks to their one-sidedness (usually intellectual) and psychological blindness."[149])

One consequence of Kafka's possession by the Sophia-anima

was that his emotional development was short-circuited. It was as if he had been seduced by a "false bride," a term used in the psychological interpretation of fairytales to describe a seductive anima figure who lures a man into the fantasy realm, away from timely responsibilities in the outside world. (It is "timely," for instance, for a young man to exploit his sexual powers, as it is appropriate for an older man to pay more attention to the inner life.) As a result, Kafka did not give Helen (i.e., sex) her due, nor did he meet his Mary at all until very near the end. In truth, while he yearned for Sophia, he was stuck with Eve, the mother. And the consequence of "not giving Helen her due," of course, was that his sexual urge often overwhelmed him: "Sex keeps gnawing at me, hounds me day and night, I should have to conquer fear and shame and probably sorrow too to satisfy it." (D2 203-204)

As "false bride," Kafka's muse was wilful and uncooperative, hence his literary output was meagre. He tried to canalize his libido into writing, but it was a constant struggle, in terms of wresting the necessary energy from the mother-complex. This phenomenon — i.e., lack of energy — is particularly common in adolescence. As Jung observes:

> The mother apparently possesses the libido of the son (the treasure she guards so jealously), and this is in fact true so long as the son remains unconscious of himself. In psychological terms this means that the "treasure hard to attain" lies hidden in the mother-imago, i.e., in the unconscious.[150]

The extent to which this was true of Kafka is evident from his diaries. The following entries are representative:

*December, 1910:*  My strength no longer suffices for another sentence. (D1 39)

*November, 1911:*  No sleep for three nights, at the slightest effort to do anything my strength is completely exhausted. (D1 152)

| | |
|---|---|
| *March, 1912:* | Today burned many old, disgusting papers. (D1 250) |
| *July, 1913:* | When I say something it immediately and finally loses its importance, when I write it down it loses it too. (D1 389) |
| *March, 1914:* | I must try to rest and sleep, otherwise I am lost in every respect. What an effort to keep alive! Erecting a monument does not require the expenditure of so much strength. (D2 23) |
| *November, 1914:* | I can't write anymore. I've come up against the last boundary, before which I shall in all likelihood sit down for years, and then in all likelihood begin another story all over again that will again remain unfinished. This fate pursues me. (D2 98) |
| *March, 1915:* | A page now and then is successful, but I can't keep it up, the next day I am powerless. (D2 116-17) |
| *December, 1915:* | I wear myself out to no purpose, should be happy if I could write, but don't. Haven't been able to get rid of my headaches lately. I have really wasted my strength away. (D2 144) |

And note this masterful image of emptiness: "Incapable of writing a line . . . . Hollow as a clamshell on the beach, ready to be pulverized by the tread of a foot." (D2 119)

\*

Kafka recorded a dream in 1911, when he was 28 years old, in which the condition of his anima is stated in no uncertain terms:

> The horrible apparition last night of a blind child, apparently the daughter of my aunt in Leitmeritz who, however, has no daughter but only sons, one of whom once broke his leg. On the other hand, there were resemblances between this child and Dr. M.'s daughter who, as I have recently seen, is in the process of changing from a pretty child into a stout, stiffly

dressed little girl. This blind or weak-sighted child had both
eyes covered by a pair of eye-glasses, the left, under a lens
held at a certain distance from the eye, was milky-grey and
bulbous, the other receded and was covered by a lens lying
close against it.

In order that this eyeglass might be set in place with op-
tical correctness it was necessary, instead of the usual support going back of the ears, to make use of a lever, the head
of which could be attached no place but to the cheekbone,
so that from this lens a little rod descended to the cheek,
there disappeared into the pierced flesh and ended on the
bone, while another small wire rod came out and went back
over the ear. (D1 74)

Notes following the dream give his associations:

I remembered that the eyeglasses in the dream derive from
my mother, who in the evening sits next to me and while
playing cards looks across at me not very pleasantly under
her eyeglasses. Her eyeglasses even have, which I do not
remember having noticed before, the right lens nearer the
eye than the left.

The child is a well-known symbol of potential future, a female
child in a man's dreams personifying his undeveloped feminine
side. Here the child is associated with an aunt who has only two
sons: the dreamer "sees" a feminine figure where in reality there
are only masculine ones. This, and the fact that if the girl really
existed she would be the sister of the aunt's son who "once broke
his leg," links the immature anima with a shadow figure who is
injured in his standpoint — just as in the later dream where the
foot of the "natural man" was tortured. (Shadow and anima
often appear in dreams as brother and sister, or married, when
contents of the unconscious are insufficiently differentiated.)

The association with Dr. M.'s pubescent daughter, changing
from a pretty girl into one "stout" and "stiffly dressed," suggests that the prognosis for her development to womanhood

through the crucial *rite de passage* of puberty is not good.

The eyes are often called the "windows of the soul"; the left eye in particular is commonly associated with the moon and Eros consciousness (relatedness through feeling).[151] Here the left eye is swollen, "milky-grey and bulbous," suggesting sickness and contamination with the mother principle. (Grey is a neutral colour, the colour of ashes and death; in Spanish and Portuguese the word for grey also means ashes.) The right eye, on the other hand, symbolizing Logos or sun consciousness, seems to be concave, i.e., receding from the light of day. In both areas there are deficiencies, the eyeglasses representing an attempt to compensate the poor vision, which itself symbolizes a lack of conscious understanding. The complicated apparatus set up to improve the sight, with the lever arrangement piercing the flesh of the cheekbone, presents a picture of facial mutilation.

Altogether, it is hardly a healthy image — not an anima figure to take one into life, nor yet one to fulfill her complementary function as mediatrix between consciousness and the unconscious.

It is interesting to note that the lens over the right eye is stabilized by a wire fixed to the cheekbone. The cheek partakes of the symbolism of the jaw, which (like the knee) was associated by the Greeks with generation and fertility.[152] The jaw also has connotations of masculine power — Samson killed a thousand Philistines with the jawbone of an ass. What is suggested here, then, is an attempt to correct the vision, the conscious attitude, by anchoring the glasses in firm masculinity.

Kafka's association of the blind child's eyeglasses with those of his mother (a connection picked up by the unconscious but not consciously noticed before) points directly to the problem: the anima is infantile, not yet a woman, because she is still tied up with the mother-imago; moreover, it is precisely this non-differentiation of his personal anima figure from the mother-imago that "blinds" Kafka's feelings.

The feeling function, as Jung describes it, evaluates, judges; it separates the wheat from the chaff. Kafka's major conflict at the time of this dream was between his writing and his job and work in his father's factory. Kafka "felt" their incompatibility, but he took no action. This is tantamount to not taking the feelings seriously. Under these conditions it is no wonder the anima "lost her sight" and therefore did not function effectively.

The mutilation involved in the attempt to compensate the anima's blindness illustrates both the tremendous effort it was for Kafka to adapt his conscious attitude to collective values (e.g., work in the "real "world), and the injury it meant to his soul.

Adaptation to collective values involves not only the ego (through ego-ideals) but also the persona, "the functional complex that comes into existence for reasons of [social] adaptation or convenience."[153] The anima, as the mediating function between the ego and the unconscious, is thus complementary to the persona, and stands in a compensatory relationship to it. That is to say, the anima reacts to the persona; a man too closely identified with his persona, his public face, will invariably experience capricious moods — the anima's compensatory attempt to bring him back to himself, as distinct from his collective role. Thus in Kafka the "injury to his soul" was a direct consequence of his attachment to persona values that were, for him, not appropriate. Psychologically speaking, there is no difference between persona identification and anima possession; both are symptoms of unconsciousness, a lack of perspective on who — and what — one really is.

The fact that Kafka's anima was so closely associated with his mother, a strong-willed, independent, and opinionated woman, manifested concretely in his attraction to women with similar qualities, i.e., women with a strong masculine side. Both Felice Bauer and Milena Jesenska fit this category, according to Max Brod. (His mother may also have been the model for the strong, dominant, sometimes overpowering female characters in his novels: women like Clara, the hotel manageress, and Brunelda in

*Amerika*; Fraulein Bürstner and Leni in *The Trial*: and Gisa and Frieda in *The Castle.*)

Such relationships may be seen as a form of compensation for Kafka's own lack of maleness. This regularly happens: the macho, "he"-man, falls for the "she"-woman, the submissive dependent female; while the sensitive, artistic, more effeminate man is irresistably drawn to the strong, masculine woman. On the other hand, it must be said that Kafka's inability fo commit himself to either of these two — Felice and Milena — suggests not only the "provisionality" and indecisiveness characteristic of the *puer,* but also a healthy resistance to "marrying his own weakness."

In the end, for the last year of his life, Kafka did establish an apparently conflict-free relationship with a woman, one who was moreover particularly feminine. This is an indication that his anima-complex, long crippled by its attachment to the mother, did finally develop — perhaps in spite of Kafka himself.

In the meantime, because Kafka lived predominantly in his head, inadequately related to his feeling side, the anima remained cool and distant, more a mother than a muse, less a friend than a jealous lover. A diary entry in August, 1917 — analogous to his note that "sex keeps gnawing at me, hounds me day and night" — shows clearly the anima's rapacious response to his conscious attitude:

> "No, let me alone! No, let me alone!" I shouted without
> pause all the way along the streets, and again and again
> she laid hold of me, again and again the clawed hands of
> the siren struck at my breast from the side or across my
> shoulder. (D2 182)

## ALIENATION AND THE ABANDONED CHILD

The psychological rule is that anything unconscious is experienced, through the process of projection, in the outside world. "When an inner situation is not made conscious," writes Jung, "it happens outside, as fate."[154]

Kafka's inner situation was alienation from himself — i.e., lack of communication with his "other side," whether seen as anima, shadow, or any other unconscious content. This lack was projected into the outside world, manifesting in a sense of alienation from his surroundings. As one critic observes:

> The total impression of his life, personality and work is that
> of a stranger alone in a world neither he nor anyone else has
> made, and which apparently has played no part in making
> him.[155]

Kafka's plight in real life was similar to that of the "hero" K. in his last novel, *The Castle* (written 1921-22). In the novel, the riddle as to why K. cannot make himself at home in the village is not solved. "K. is a stranger," notes Max Brod, "and has struck a village in which strangers are looked upon with suspicion."[156]

Here again there is a projection into the outside world of Kafka's attitude towards himself: his feelings of inferiority and obsession with perfection meant he could never be "good" enough to merit friendship and respect; because he could not live up to his ego ideals and expectations of himself, he looked upon himself with "suspicion." In short, he was haunted by the possibility that his life — like that of Tolstoi's Ivan Ilyich, but for precisely opposite reasons — had been unproductive, a waste of time. Speaking to Gustav Janouch of his "imprisonment," he said:

> Everything looks as if it were made of solid, lasting stuff. But
> on the contrary it is a life in which one is falling towards an
> abyss. But if one closes one's eyes, one can hear its rush and
> roar.[157]

For Ivan Ilyich, a public official like Kafka, it was the life-long indifference to his inner life that on his death-bed drove him to despair. For Kafka, it was the fear that he had concentrated on himself too much:

> A little story I read today revived in me the long unheeded, ever present question of whether the cause of my downfall was not insane selfishness, mere anxiety for self; not, moreover, anxiety for a higher self, but vulgar anxiety for my well-being. (D2 222)

From a strictly materialistic point of view, there is some truth in this self-accusation, in that Kafka opted to founder in a half-life because his existence would indeed have been financially precarious had he devoted all his time and energy to writing. But from a psychological point of view one might say that he was actually not selfish enough. By this I mean he did not take seriously enough his own feelings and emotional reactions — again and again he sided with collective values, against himself, in terms of what he "should" be, "ought to" do, etc., instead of how he really felt.

It is not that his aspirations in the social community were misguided per se; they simply didn't work for him. A productive relationship with the outside world has to be based on a healthy working relationship with oneself. First things first; charity begins at home — charity towards the conflicting, childish, autonomous elements within oneself. To call this "vulgar anxiety" for one's "well-being" is another symptom of negative inflation; it leads directly to guilt, self-denigration, and masochistic suffering. Moreover, since the unconscious is, as the collective psyche, the psychological representative of society, to be in touch with it actually brings one closer to others.

Alienation from the unconscious is commonly experienced as not being part of the group. "I'm always an outsider," complains the misfit, "I can always think of some reason why I don't fit in. I stand on the edge of the group and wish I were like everyone else." This is another characteristic lament of the *puer*, deriving from the secret, or completely unconscious, belief that he is really superior, somebody special. Of course it is the other, compensatory face of inflation, and the best antidote to it is the realization and acceptance of one's shadow side, and ordinary humanity; i.e., the instincts, which are common to everyone.

Subjectively, alienation is closely identified with the feeling of being "abandoned," a condition mythologically associated with the childhood of gods and divine heroes (Zeus, Dionysus, Poseidon, Moses, Romulus and Remus, etc.). In fact so widespread is this motif that Jung describes abandonment as "a necessary condition and not just a concomitant symptom" of the potentially higher consciousness symbolized by the child[158] — for instance when it appears in dreams.

Anyone in the process of becoming independent must of necessity detach himself from his origins, both familial and societal — not necessarily physically, but certainly psychologically. This involves, in the broadest terms, differentiating oneself from the collective. The result is two-fold: the "poor me" syndrome characteristic of the childish, regressive longing for dependence, and a certain psychic experience of a creative nature — the positive side of the divine child (*puer aeternus*) archetype. Jung writes:

> In the psychology of the individual there is always, at such moments, an agonizing situation of conflict from which there seems to be no way out — at least for the conscious mind, since as far as this is concerned, *tertium non datur.*[159]

That is to say, the *tertium*, the "third" that would resolve the conflict between the opposites (in this case oneself and the collective) is not logically accessible to consciousness. It rests rather with the unconscious to come up with a solution, namely an attitude of mind that is better adapted to oneself and one's circumstances.

The suffering engendered by the conflict is the price that has to be paid in order to grow up, and initially it goes hand in hand

with the subjective experience of loneliness — behind which is
the archetypal motif of the abandoned child. Thus Jung observes:

> Higher consciousness, or knowledge going beyond our present-
> day consciousness, is equivalent to being *all alone in the world.*
> This loneliness expresses the conflict between the bearer or
> symbol of higher consciousness and his surroundings.[160]

Kafka's loneliness had in fact both these elements: the "poor
me" syndrome, neatly expressed in the "secret raven" passage
already quoted — a most literary way of saying, "Nobody suffers as much as I do"; and isolation from his contemporaries by
a vision of reality quite out of the ordinary.

Psychologically the sense of loneliness and isolation indicates
a lack of, and therefore need for, communication with the various personalities within oneself, i.e., personifications of complexes. The individual psyche is peopled, so to speak, with potential
companions. (Recall Kafka's dream in 1914, ending: "Some man,
a shadow, a companion, is always at my side.") Further, loneliness can spring not only from the neglect of, for instance,
anima/animus and shadow (Kafka: "I don't know who it is.
Really have no time to turn around, to turn sideways"), but also
from the abandonment of one's own inner child, one's potential
future.

The child in oneself cannot grow unless and until it is cared for.
This applies to both aspects of the child: the childish — manifesting in emotional immaturity and the provisional life — and the
childlike — appearing as spontaneity, creativity, and openness to
change. The former is to be accepted in hopes that it will mature;
the latter is to be cultivated in order that life have some meaning.
It is seldom easy to determine, in any particular situation, which
aspect of the child is involved; but embracing the inherent ambivalence of one's own psychology is often the step that trans-
forms the conscious, ego attitude, releasing new energy. It is this
point that Kafka may finally have won through to. "Eternal
childhood," he notes in October, 1921. "Life calls again."
(D2 195)

With this in mind, Kafka's life-long conflicts may be seen as a consequence of his resistance to both aspects of his own child: he was ashamed of his "dependence," and he deplored the responsibility and sacrifices involved in nurturing his creative talent. His intense longing for children, then (recall: "The infinite, deep, warm, saving happiness of sitting beside the cradle of one's child opposite its mother"), would be a compensatory reaction to his failure to accept this fundamental inner responsibility, and therefore symbolic of his need for psychic rebirth — i.e., a new attitude. Indeed, Kafka himself said as much, albeit unwittingly:

> Outwardly, I fulfil my duties satisfactorily in the office, not my inner duties, however, and every unfulfilled inner duty becomes a misfortune that never leaves. (D1 59)

Furthermore, the "mother" Kafka looked for in vain in the outside world, the woman who would bear his children, is one of the psychological functions of the anima. Kafka's real task was thus to impregnate his soul — by paying more attention to it — and this, at least until near the end of his life, he failed to do. The tragedy in these terms, then, is that he sought outside what can only be found within.

Kafka's psychological situation, and its potential solution, was, again, succinctly pictured by Kafka himself in one of his fragments, called "A Little Fable":

> "Alas," said the mouse, "the world is growing smaller every day. At the beginning it was so big that I was afraid, I kept running and running, and I was glad when at last I saw walls far away to the right and left, but these long walls have narrowed so quickly that I am in the last chamber already, and there in the corner stands the trap that I must run into."
>
> "You only need to change direction," said the cat, and ate it up.[161]

Here the cat appears as a symbol for the mother-complex, the imprisoning "trap" that effectively prevented Kafka (as a mouse instead of a man) from "changing direction," that is, reorienting his conscious attitude.

## 4 TRANSFORMATION

Kafka's published diaries end in June, 1923 — a year before he died — with the following entry:

> More and more fearful as I write. It is understandable. Every word, twisted in the hands of the spirits — this twist of the hand is their characteristic gesture — becomes a spear turned against the speaker. Most especially a remark like this. And so ad infinitum. The only consolation would be: it happens whether you like or not. And what you like is of infinitesimally little help. More than consolation is: You too have weapons. (D2 233)

A final note of quiet desperation, the fear of "every word" indicating his continuing struggle to assimilate the male, "father" world (society, Logos, the Word); while the spear "turned against" him suggests an intuition turned negative[162] — and possibly also a touch of paranoia.

Such expressions of despair are so rife in Kafka's diaries that the danger exists of accepting his pessimism as absolute, his life as "nothing but" one of sorrow and unrelieved misery. Yet, as he declares in that last diary entry, he too had "weapons." Indeed, in my opinion he had only two: one was his writing, the other was the thin thread of hope running through his life. As he writes in February, 1915:

> If I were another person observing myself and the course of my life, I should be compelled to say that it must all end unavailingly, be consumed in incessant doubt, creative only in its self-torment. But, an interested party, I go on hoping. (D2 116)

And in truth, his hope was fulfilled, for in July, 1923, at the age of 40, almost immediately after his last diary entry, he met the young girl Dora Dymant and his life changed dramatically.

It is my feeling that this was a synchronistic event, meaning it was something Kafka was "ready" for — a "chance" meeting in the outside world that coincided with the inner development of his anima. In psychological terms, Dora Dymant represented the resolution of the ego-shadow conflict through the aegis of the feminine.[163]

Appropriately enough, Kafka found his "soul-mate" scaling fish in a kitchen.[164] What better place to find an anima figure than in a kitchen — the centre of the house, the alchemical "laboratory," the place of transformation? And what more propitious occupation for her than cleaning fish — a symbol of (to name but a few) *fertility* (Ishtar, Oannes), *sexuality* (Osiris, Aphrodite), *resurrection and immortality* (Osiris, Christ, Noah), *salvation* (Vishnu, the Rabbinical Messiah, Christ, Pisces), *wisdom* (Oannes, Varuna), *the beginning of all things* (Tiamat, Leviathan), *wholeness* (the *lapis* in alchemy), *healing* (Tobias in The Book of Tobit), and *redemption through suffering* (Christ).[165] In short, the fish is a symbol of renewal and rebirth, precisely what Dora Dymant herself meant to Kafka.

According to Max Brod, there was no hesitation, no conflict:

> His decision to cut all ties, get to Berlin, and live with Dora stood firm — and this time he carried it out inflexibly. At the end of July he left Prague, after offering successful resistance to all his family's objections. From Berlin he wrote to me for the first time that he felt happy, and that he was even sleeping well — an unheard-of novelty in these last years.[166]

And so at last Kafka made a commitment; he knew what he wanted and directed all his energies towards getting it. That is the masculine way par excellence. Brod visited the couple in Berlin and found "an idyll":

> At last I saw my friend in good spirits; his bodily health had got worse, it is true. Yet for the time being it was not even

dangerous. Franz spoke about the demons which had at last
let go of him. "I have slipped away from them. This moving
to Berlin was magnificent, now they are looking for me and
can't find me, at least for the moment."[167]

Kafka had finally achieved his ideal of an independent life, a
home of his own; no longer was he a son living with his parents,
but to a certain extent was himself the head of a family. And
his last few months were by all accounts, including his own
letters, not only the happiest period of his life but one of the
most creative as well.[168]

I am not concerned here with that last year of Kafka's life. The
period is well covered in Max Brod's biography, including a very
moving account of Kafka's last few days. I am interested rather
in what had been constellated in Kafka, preceding his "chance"
encounter with Dora Dymant, to make it possible. What had happened to the indecisive, melancholic, dependent neurotic who
at the height of his despair in 1920 wrote: "Some deny the existence of misery by pointing to the sun; he denies the existence
of the sun by pointing to misery"?[169]

It is Jung's view that a neurosis, especially in the second half
of life, is never "cured" without the development of a religious
attitude. "The term 'religion,' " writes Jung, "designates the attitude peculiar to a consciousness which has been changed by experience of the *numinosum*."[170] Elsewhere he declares that a
man in a conflict situation has to rely on

> divine comfort and mediation . . . . an autonomous psychic
> happening, a hush that follows the storm, a reconciling light
> in the darkness . . . secretly bringing order into the chaos of
> his soul.[171]

This is what seems to have happened to Kafka — but it is not
what is usually meant when he is referred to as a "religious"
writer. His reputation in that respect is based on his work as a
search for meaning. For Kafka preached no particular dogma,
nor was he a "believer" in any conventional sense. His "religi-

osity" was in fact quite as compatible with atheism as with a belief in God.[172]

But psychologically, Jung's use (and mine here) of the terms
"religious" and "religious attitude" implies something rather different; namely, an attitude of mind based on an experience of
transcendental reality, the *reality of the psyche.* With this goes
an attitude that acknowledges the presence of autonomous gods
within, in other words archetypal contents to which the ego itself is subordinate and must pay heed.

Good psychic health is in this sense a gift of the gods — the
gods within. And from this point of view neurosis might be characterized as a sign that the gods within are not pleased — an un-
pleasant condition to live through, but teleologically an excellent
basis for hope. This is to say that neurosis is by no means all negative, a point Jung emphasized in his Tavistock lectures:

> *Dr. Dicks:* I understand, then, that the outbreak of a neurot-
> ic illness, from the point of view of man's development, is
> something favourable?
>
> *Professor Jung:* That is so . . . . That is really my point of
> view. I am not altogether pessimistic about neurosis. In many
> cases we have to say: "Thank heaven he could make up his
> mind to be neurotic." Neurosis is really an attempt at self-
> cure, just as any physical disease is part an attempt at self-
> cure . . . . [Neurosis] is an attempt of the self-regulating psy-
> chic system to restore the balance, in no way different from
> the function of dreams — only rather more forceful and dras-
> tic.[173]

For many years, then, Kafka's inner gods were not pleased.
Work, marriage, family — each new setback in the outside world
drove him further into himself, where he perpetuated the anguish
of self-analysis. "This inescapable duty to observe oneself," he
writes in November, 1921. "If someone else is observing me,
naturally I have to observe myself too; if no one observes me, I
have to observe myself all the closer." (D2 200) In terms of inner

change, however, the evidence suggests that the period October, 1921, to March, 1922, was decisive.

That was a particularly bad time for Kafka. Years of frustration lay behind him; he was in the process of ending the painful liaison with Milena; his health was rapidly deteriorating; he had written nothing for months. But in spite of the continuing despair and depression — perhaps even because of it — there is every indication in the diaries of what amounts to a psychological breakthrough. It is a climax of sorts, the culmination of holding the tension of all his conflicts all those years, and it did involve an experience of the *numinosum*, the reality of the psyche.

On October 20, 1921, Kafka had the following dream:

> A short dream, during an agitated, short sleep, in agitation clung to it with a feeling of boundless happiness. A dream with many ramifications, full of a thousand connections that become clear in a flash; but hardly more than a basic mood remains:
>
> My brother had committed a crime, a murder, I think, I and other people were involved in the crime; punishment, solution and salvation approached from afar, loomed up powerfully, many signs indicated their ineluctable approach; my sister, I think, kept calling out these signs as they appeared and I kept greeting them with insane exclamations, brief sentences merely, because of their succinctness, and now don't clearly remember a single one.
>
> I could only have uttered brief exclamations because of the great effort it cost me to speak — I had to puff out my cheeks and at the same time contort my mouth as if I had a toothache before I could bring a word out. My feeling of happiness lay in the fact that I welcomed so freely, with such conviction and such joy, the punishment that came, a sight that must have moved the gods, and I felt the gods' emotion almost to the point of tears. (D2 196-197)

"My brother had committed a crime, a murder." Kafka had no brothers (two died in infancy, when he was a child), so we may take this as a shadow figure. That he commits a crime means, psychologically, that the ego has relinquished action to the un- conscious — forced the shadow to be the man, as it were (as Cain had to take on the responsibility, so to speak, for the first mur- der). Murder is the most serious crime, showing the extent to which the aggressive, masculine instincts are unconscious.

At the same time, "I and other people were involved in the crime," indicating that the ego cannot altogether escape respon- sibility for what happens "unconsciously" (a logical consequence of the compensatory function of the unconscious). The "punish- ment, solution and salvation" seems to herald a release of inner tension — though it is still some distance away ("afar" meaning deep in the collective unconscious).

The sister in the dream no doubt refers to Kafka's favourite sister Ottilie, with whom he lived at times. Five years earlier he described his feelings about her:

> At times Ottilie seems to me to be what I should want a
> mother to be: pure, truthful, honest, consistent. Humility
> and pride, sympathetic understanding and distance, devo-
> tion and independence, vision and courage in unerring bal-
> ance. I mention Ottilie because Mother is in her too, though
> it is impossible to discern. (D2 168)

As an inner anima figure, then, although still connected with the mother, she is considerably more positive than the blind child in Kafka's dream of October, 1911. In fact it is generally true that a "sister-anima" represents an advance in a man's emotional development, a stage midway between Eve (the mother) and Helen (sex).

In the dream Kafka is virtually speechless: "I had to puff out my cheeks . . . as if I had a toothache."

Swollen cheeks bring to mind the representation of the winds on old maps, echoed in Shakespeare's lines, "To tear with thun- der the wide cheeks o' th' air" (Coriolanus 5,3) and "Blow, winds, and crack your cheeks" (King Lear 3, 2:5). Wind itself, in many

religious and mythological connections (Pentecost, the Hebraic
rûah, Marduk vs. Chaos, Gilgamesh vs. Humbaba), represents the
creative spirit (hence "inspiration"); thus the forceful effort to
speak may compensate a conscious lack of creative energy.

Teeth, through Perseus's mythological theft of the Graea's one
tooth, are associated with power. Teeth falling out, or broken,
in dreams frequently point to a real situation in which one is
"losing one's grip." Teeth are also connected with wisdom (the
Celtic hero Fionn placed his thumb under his tooth whenever
he needed guidance) and fertility (e.g., the legends that men were
born of snakes' teeth planted in the ground).[174] The "toothache,"
then, suggests a degree of impotence, which is itself associated
with childhood. Psychologically this would indicate the need to
grow up, as in Jung's remark: "Anyone who does not understand
the events that befall him is always in danger of getting stuck in
the transitional stage [Father-Son-Holy Ghost] of the Son."[175]

In terms of Kafka at the time, the aggressiveness of the shadow
"brother," clamouring for attention by committing murder,
would compensate both a conscious suppression of Kafka's "natural man" and his decidedly passive, non-violent nature. (In the
Letter to His Father, Kafka describes himself as "weakly, timid,
hesitant"[176]; Brod agrees: "And what was there that Franz lack-
ed more than push?"[177])

The attempt to speak certainly compensates Kafka's lack of
creative drive in reality, and the forgetfulness of the "signs" indicates that consciously he is not yet ready to assimilate the information coming up. On the other hand, the fact that the sister-
anima functions here positively, as mediatrix between the dream
ego and the "signs" approaching from the deep unconscious,
strongly suggests a conscious attitude more receptive than hitherto.

The feeling-tone of a dream is always particularly important.
Here there is a feeling of happiness due to the possibility of salvation through punishment (similar to the motif of redemption

through suffering — past, present, and yet to come), while the joyful acceptance by Kafka of his fate apparently pleases the gods too — the gods within. (A few months later Kafka writes: "Told M. about the night, unsatisfactory. Accept your symptoms, don't complain of them; immerse yourself in your suffering." — D2 209. This is to say, in effect, "care for your own child," and "keep the vessel closed.")

The overall impression is that this dream presages something extraordinary "in the wind" (swollen cheeks!) for Kafka. But meanwhile, since the shadow still has all the energy (and so in a sense it is the ego that has been murdered), ego-consciousness would experience a loss of libido, i.e., depression.

And in fact the diary entries over the next few months reflect prolonged moods of despair. Again there is the image of a prison:

> All is imaginary — family, office, friends, the street, all imaginary, far away or close at hand, the woman; the truth that lies closest, however, is only this, that you are beating your head against the wall of a windowless and doorless cell. (D2 197)

In January, 1922, he writes: "Fretful that my life till now has been merely marking time, has progressed at most in the sense that decay progresses in a rotten tooth" (D2 209) — another indication of continuing powerlessness. And in March:

> How would it be if one were to choke to death on oneself? If the pressure of introspection were to diminish, or close off entirely, the opening through which one flows forth into the world? I am not far from it at times. A river flowing upstream. For a long time now, that is what for the most part has been going on. (D2 223)

Kafka's libido was absolutely blocked. It could not flow "forth into the world," so it backed up: "a river flowing upstream." This extraordinary image of the backward flow of energy shows the *contra naturam* aspect of the developmental process. It is apparently "against nature" to become conscious, and it frequently looks and feel like regression. But the movement "upstream," to the source (i.e., the unconscious), is often a necessary stage in development in the sense of *reculer pour mieux sauter* — a move backwards, the better to leap ahead. As Jung observes:

> By activating an unconscious factor, regression confronts consciousness with the problem of the psyche as opposed to the problem of outward adaptation. It is natural that the conscious mind should fight against accepting the regressive contents, yet it is finally compelled by the impossibility of further progress to submit to the regressive values. In other words, regression leads to the necessity of adapting to the inner world of the psyche.[178]

This would explain, in Kafka's case, why his suffering this time, rather than self-indulgent or masochistic, was ultimately meaningful.

Nevertheless, the outer face of this process is initially depression, and during this period of Kafka's life there was nothing to break the inward spiral of unproductive activity. Everything, wherever he went, pointed up with relentless insistence his inability to take part in the most ordinary social activities:

> Incapable of striking up a friendship with anyone, incapable of tolerating a friendship, at bottom full of endless astonishment when I see a group of people cheerfully assembled together. (D2 214)

A walk in the park, the sight of laughing couples, torments him unbearably:

> I do not envy particular married couples, I simply envy all married couples together; and even when I do envy one couple only, it is the happiness of married life in general, in all its infinite variety, that I envy — the happiness to be found in any one marriage, even in the likeliest case, would probably plunge me into despair. (D2 195)

Or, alternatively:

> No envy. Enough imagination to share their happiness, enough
> judgement to know that I am too weak to have such happiness,
> foolish enough to think I see to the bottom of my own and
> their situation. Not foolish enough; there is a tiny crack there,
> the wind whistles through it and spoils the full effect. (D2 194)

The "denouement," as Kafka describes it, came in January,
1922. Early in the month he suffered "something very like a
breakdown," which he interprets in two ways, "both of which
are probably correct":

> First: breakdown, impossible to sleep, impossible to stay
> awake, impossible to endure life, or, more exactly, the course
> of life. The clocks are not in unison; the inner one runs crazi-
> ly on at a devilish or demoniac or in any case inhuman pace,
> the outer one limps along at its usual speed. What else can
> happen but that the two worlds split apart, and they do split
> apart, or at least clash in a fearful manner. There are doubt-
> less several reasons for the wild tempo of the inner process;
> the most obvious one is introspection, which will suffer no
> idea to sink tranquilly to rest but must pursue each one into
> consciousness, only itself to become an idea, in turn to be
> pursued by renewed introspection.
>
> Second: This pursuit, originating in the midst of men,
> carries one in a direction away from them. The solitude that
> for the most part has been forced on me, in part voluntarily
> sought by me — but what was this if not compulsion too? —
> is now losing all its ambiguity and approaches its denouement.
> Where is it leading? The strongest likelihood is that it may
> lead to madness; there is nothing more to say, the pursuit
> goes right through me and rends me asunder. (D2 202)

This clearly illustrates the degree to which Kafka's "two worlds"
had become polarized, resulting in a "mid-life crisis." The tension and disharmony were greater than ever ("the clocks are not
in unison"), hence all his libido turned inward, seeking rebirth

from the source. Subjectively it was a monumental depression; psychologically it was regression; but teleologically it was a necessary phase in his development. As Jung notes:

> The individual is . . . not consciously aware that he is developing; he feels himself to be in a compulsive situation that resembles an early infantile state or even an embryonic condition within the womb. It is only if he remains stuck in this condition that we can speak of involution or degeneration.[179]

Kafka did not remain stuck. Rather the pressure continued to mount, and a series of diary entries at the end of January suggests that something unexpected (the *tertium non datur*, the "third" not logically given) was approaching consciousness. On the 18th he writes:

> A moment of thought: Resign yourself, learn (learn, forty-year-old) to rest content in the moment (yes, once you could do it). Yes, in the moment, in the terrible moment. It is not so terrible, only your fear of the future makes it so.  (D2 203)

On the 19th:

> Evil does not exist; once you have crossed the threshhold, all is good. Once in another world, you must hold your tongue.
> (D2 205)

And on the 20th:

> As in the despairing hour of death you cannot meditate on right and wrong, so you cannot in the despairing hour of life. It is enough that the arrows fit exactly in the wounds that they have made.  (D2 206)

Symbolically, the arrows are the projections of himself into the outside world, the ego-illusions and false expectations he maintained for years; now (to mix a metaphor) they are coming home to roost, a painful but unavoidable step in the process of "grounding," that is, growing up. Alternatively (or as well), the arrows may be seen as introverting libido, due to the denial of the instincts. "The wounding and painful shafts," writes Jung, "do not come from outside . . . but from the ambush of our own unconscious. It is our own repressed desires that stick like arrows in our flesh."[180]

At last, on January 28th, there is calm and a sense of peaceful acceptance. He writes:

> I am now a citizen of this other world, whose relationship to the ordinary one is the relationship of the wilderness to cultivated land (I have been forty years wandering from Canaan); I look back at it like a foreigner, though in this other world as well — it is the parental heritage I carry with me — I am the most insignificant and timid of all creatures and am able to keep alive thanks only to the special nature of its arrangements.  (D2 213)

It is apparent from this that Kafka had weathered the storm; in some rationally inexplicable fashion he had come to terms with himself. He continues:

> In this world it is possible even for the humblest to be raised to the heights as if with lightning speed, though they can also be crushed forever as if by the weight of the seas.  (D2 213)

— a striking image, analogous to the "clashing rocks" motif of heroic, funerary, and shamanic mythologies in different parts of the world. In initiation rituals and folklore this dangerous or paradoxical passage to the "other side" is envisioned variously as clashing rocks; dancing, razor-sharp reeds; snapping jaws of monstrous animals; opening and closing waters (e.g., the flight of the Jews from Egypt into the Promised Land); shifting islands (or, among the Eskimos, icebergs); and other versions of the classic Symplegades (rocks) that threatened to crush the Argonauts. Among the Huichol Indians, the "dangerous passage" is called "The Gateway of the Clashing Clouds."[181] These are all concretizations of a psychic process that is inherently risky. Sensibly, then, Kafka adds:

> Should I not be thankful despite everything? Was it certain that I should find my way to this world? Could not "banishment" from one side, coming together with rejection from this, have crushed me at the border?  (D2 213)

Kafka's "banishment," of course, like his imprisonment, was psychological, an attitude of mind, and only as a committed "citizen of this other world" (the inner one) did there exist for Kafka the real possibility of satisfaction in the outer one. Now it was only a matter of time until "outer mirrored inner" — in the person of Dora Dymant.

Particularly significant is the fact that Kafka's "subjective experience . . . of a religious order," his apprehension of "the reality of the psyche," was not a matter of blinding lights or fireworks, nor was it a momentary revelation of heavenly bliss. It was rather a solid, experiential realization of his own reality, as real as hard rock, as real as "the weight of the seas," — and as such, it changed his conscious attitude.

Nor is it without significance that this happened in the midst of Kafka's 40th year. The number 40 is enormously numinous in Judaic-Christian tradition, involved as it is in *anticipation* (Moses on the Mount for 40 days; Israel in the wilderness 40 years; Christ in the tomb 40 hours before resurrection, and on earth 40 days before ascension); *punishment and purification* (40 days of rain for the flood, after another 40 Noah opened the window; Elijah in the desert, fed by ravens, for 40 days; Christ's 40 days fasting in the desert, hence 40 days of Lent; in alchemy the *lapis* appears in the retort after 40 days); and *maturity* (at 40 a man is supposed to be "ripe" — Genesis 25:20, 26:34, Joshua 4:7; Moses' life was divided into three periods of 40 years each; Esau and Isaac married at 40). In addition, there are 40 weeks of human pre-natal existence in the womb.[182] It was perhaps with some or all of this in mind that Kafka himself noted (above): "I have been forty years wandering from Canaan."

Not that the remaining diary entries (only a handful of pages) are all sunshine and roses. "Unnoticeable life. Noticeable failure," he writes on February 20, 1922. (D2 223) On March 7: "Yesterday the worst night I have had; as if everything were at an end." (D2 223) Yet they lack the desperate bite of those before the turning point. For one thing, they seem to derive more from the physical pain of his tuberculosis than from psychological distress. For another, the complaints are relieved by observations of a happier tone. February 2: "The happiness of being with people." (D2 218) February 13: "The possibility of serving with all one's might." (D2 222) And on February 26:

> I grant . . . that possibilities exist in me, possibilities close at
> hand that I don't yet know of; only to find the way to them!
> and when I have found it, to dare!  (D2 223)

On the whole, these last few entries suggest that although Kafka wasn't yet out of the woods (that is, the mother-complex), he was at least moving in that direction. This feeling is reinforced by a close look at a dream he had on March 23, 1922:

> In the afternoon dreamed of the boil on my cheek. The per-
> petually shifting frontier that lies between ordinary life and
> the terror that would seem to be more real.  (D2 225)

Biblical references to boils show them as an indication of God's displeasure; e.g., as the sixth sign of Moses in Egypt, where ashes sprinkled "toward heaven in the sight of the Pharaoh" became "small dust in all the land of Egypt, and shall be a boil breaking forth with blains upon men" (Exodus 9:8,9); and as one of the afflictions visited upon Job: "So went Satan forth from the presence of the Lord, and smote Job with sore boils from the sole of his foot unto his crown." (Job 2:7)

But painful as they are, boils also serve to bring to the surface the poison within; i.e., they rid the system of destructive elements. In this sense they are like a depression, which can activate unconscious contents and bring them to the light of day. The boil is then a physical manifestation (he actually had one) of what Kafka had experienced during the previous few months. It might be noted, too, that among primitive peoples the skin in general is equated with the soul; and skin diseases, in all past ages and cultures, in all parts of the world, have ever been regarded as a visitation from God or the devil (again, the idea of "gods within").[183]

The cheek is perhaps the least individual part of the face, so we may suspect that the "poison" originates in a more collective attitude or aspect of life. Psychologically, this would relate to the persona ("putting on a good face") and ego-ideals. In addition, the cheek/jaw-bone, as already indicated, has traditional associations with generation, fertility, and masculinity, as well as the spirit.

Interestingly enough, these amplifications connect the boil on Kafka's cheek not only with his dream of the "blind child" anima whose face was disfigured by a wire attached to the cheekbone, and the dream of October 20, 1921 ("I had to puff out my cheeks . . ."), but also with his ass/greyhound dream of ten years earlier (which showed the spiritualization of the chthonic shadow, a consequence of Kafka's youthful ideals). Here, then, is another "thin thread" running through Kafka's life: soul and shadow "damaged" by a rigid consciousness holding on to collective values and attitudes that were personally inappropriate.

All this, it would seem, came to the surface in the boil: a lifetime of neurotic suffering due to the "blinding" of his soul; a timid, weak, retiring "provisionality" due to the rejection of his "natural man"; and an emotional immaturity that kept him dependent due to the "imprisoning" effect of the mother-complex.

Three weeks after the boil dream, on April 11, 1922, as if to sum up the effect on Kafka of the previous six months' "punishment," there is a bare-bones, two-line diary entry:

> Eternal youth is impossible; even if there were no other obstacle, introspection would make it impossible. (D2 227)

This betokens the death of childish illusions, the virtual rout of the *puer*; the way has been prepared for Kafka to become a responsible adult, a man.

# Notes

Publication details are in the Bibliography
CW — *The Collected Works of C.G. Jung*

1. Angel Flores (ed.), *The Kafka Problem*, p. ix.
2. Ibid.
3. Cf. esp. "Psychology and Literature," in *The Spirit in Man, Art and Literature*, CW 15.
4. Marie-Louise von Franz, *The Problem of the Puer Aeternus*, p. I/1.
5. "Psychology and Literature," in *The Spirit in Man, Art and Literature*, CW 15, par. 156.
6. Max Brod, *Franz Kafka, A Biography*, p. 40.
7. Ibid., p. 97.
8. Ibid., p. 96.
9. "Reflections on Sin, Pain, Hope and the True Way," in *The Great Wall of China and Other Pieces*, p. 146.
10. Gustav Janouch, *Conversations with Kafka*, p. 178.
11. The term anima, used psychologically, refers to the unconscious, feminine side of a man's personality. It is his "soul-image," which when projected onto a real woman is experienced as "falling in love." (Cf. C.G. Jung, "Definitions," in *Psychological Types*, CW 6, pars. 808-811)
12. *Letters to Milena*, p. 163.
13. *Letter to His Father*, p. 99.
14. Brod, op. cit., p. 143.
15. Ibid., p. 156.
16. Ibid., p. 217.
17. *Letters to Milena*, pp. 214-215.
18. *Letter to His Father*, p. 111.
19. Ironically, Kafka did father a child without being aware of it. The boy died suddenly in 1921, just before the age of seven. The mother, who never contacted Kafka, is thought to have shared the fate of other Jewish prisoners in Nazi concentration camps during World War II. (Cf. Brod, op. cit., pp. 240-242)
20. *Letter to His Father*, p. 113.
21. Ibid., p. 115.
22. Ibid., p. 110.
23. Ibid., p. 68.

24. Ibid., p. 69. The reference is to the last line of *The Trial*.

25. The term animus is used psychologically to mean the unconscious, masculine side of a woman's personality. It is the Logos, spirit principle in women. An "animus woman" refers to one identified with her masculine side; this manifests in rigid opinions and an argumentative attitude. (Cf. C.G. Jung, *Aion*, CW 9, II, par. 29; and *Two Essays on Analytical Psychology*, CW 7, par. 331)

26. *Letter to His Father*, p. 45.

27. Janouch, op. cit., p. 53.

28. Brod, op. cit., p. 95.

29. Ibid., p. 96.

30. "The Street Window," in *The Penal Colony*, p. 39.

31. "He" (Notes from the Year 1920), in *The Great Wall of China and Other Pieces*, p. 136.

32. Walter Kaufmann (ed.), *Nietzsche*, p. 50. The passage in full: "Thinking of oneself gives little happiness. If, however, one feels much happiness in this, it is because at bottom one is not thinking of oneself but of one's ideal. This is far, and only the swift reach it and are delighted."

33. Thomas Mann, *Tonio Kröger*, pp. 158-159.

34. Ibid., p. 190.

35. Ibid.

36. Brod, op. cit., p. 78.

37. The existence of autonomous, unconscious complexes, or "feeling-toned complexes of ideas" (because they are always accompanied by emotion), was first demonstrated scientifically by Jung in his association experiments 75 years ago. (Cf. *Experimental Researches*, CW 2) Complexes are normal and present in everyone; they are the living units of the psyche, and as such are commonly personified in dreams, drawings, and fantasies. "The *via regia* to the unconscious," writes Jung, "is not the dream, as [Freud] thought, but the complex, which is the architect of dreams and of symptoms." ("A Review of the Complex Theory," in *The Structure and Dynamics of the Psyche*, CW 8, par. 210)

38. *Mysterium Coniunctionis*, CW 14, par. 514n.

39. Jung's theory of psychological types identifies two personality attitudes, introverted and extraverted, and four basic functions: sensation, thinking, feeling, and intuition. (Cf. "Definitions," in *Psychological Types*, CW 6) In brief: *sensation* tells us that a thing exists; *thinking* tells us what it is; *feeling* tells us what it's worth to us; and *intuition* tells us

what we can do with it (the possibilities). For practical reasons it is necessary to distinguish feeling — as a rational, judgemental function — from emotion, which comes from an activated complex. (Cf. Note 37 above)

40. *Aion*, CW 9, II, par. 252.

41. Cf. especially Selma Fraiberg, "Kafka and the Dream," in Wm. Phillips (ed.), *Art and Psychoanalysis*; Walter H. Sokel, *Franz Kafka*; and Martin Greenberg, *The Terror of Art*.

42. "The Eight Octavo Notebooks and Fragments from Notebooks and Loose Pages," in *Wedding Preparations in the Country and Other Posthumous Writings*, p. 272.

43. Ibid., p. 330.

44. Ibid., p. 50.

45. Ibid., p. 148.

46. Ibid., p. 73.

47. "Reflections," in *The Great Wall of China*, p. 142.

48. This remark evokes Kafka's short story, "In the Penal Colony," in which a machine scratches the condemned man's crime on his body.

49. The psychological significance of the Grail and the symbolism associated with it, is thoroughly explored by Emma Jung and Marie-Louise von Franz in *The Grail Legend*. The most exhaustive historical and mythological study of the old king motif is J.G. Fraser's *The Golden Bough*.

50. "Definitions," in *Psychological Types*, CW 6, par. 693.

51. "Reflections," in *The Great Wall of China*, p. 142.

52. Von Franz, *The Problem of the Puer Aeternus*, p. VIII/13.

53. "The Structure of the Unconscious," in *Two Essays on Analytical Psychology*, CW 7, par. 487.

54. *The Visions Seminars*, p. 336.

55. Ibid., p. 305.

56. "Some Crucial Points in Psychoanalysis" (Jung-Loy Correspondence), in *Freud and Psychoanalysis*, CW 4, par. 606.

57. Ibid., par. 607.

58. "The Relations Between the Ego and the Unconscious," in *Two Essays on Analytical Psychology*, CW 7, par. 258.

59. "He," in *The Great Wall of China*, p. 135.

60. "The Psychology of the Transference," in *The Practice of Psychotherapy*, CW 16, par. 470.

61. *Letters to Milena*, pp. 204-205.

62. "Reflections," in *The Great Wall of China*, p. 151.

63. Cf. Jung, *Psychology and Religion*, CW 11, pars. 126, 136, and esp. 250.

64. Richard Wilhelm (transl.), *The I Ching or Book of Changes*, p. 11.

65. Brod, op. cit., pp. 39-40.

66. Ibid., p. 78.

67. Introductory Note, *The Great Wall of China*, p. 6.

68. Brod, op. cit., p. 93.

69. Walter Kaufmann (ed.), op. cit., p. 228.

70. *Letters*, Vol. 1:1906-1950, p. 375.

71. *Mysterium Coniunctionis*, CW 14, par. 514.

72. "Psychology and Religion," in *Psychology and Religion*, ( , 11, par. 9.

73. "A Psychological Approach to the Dogma of the Trinity," ibid., par. 260.

74. "Tractatus aureus," *Ars chemica*, p. 12. (Quoted by Jung in *Mysterium Coniunctionis*, CW 14, par. 37)

75. Ibid., par. 741.

76. Cf. von Franz, *A Psychological Interpretation of the Golden Ass of Apuleius*, p. 44.

77. Cf. Patricia Dale-Green, *Dog*, pp. 23-24.

78. Von Franz, *Individuation in Fairytales*, p. 86.

79. Cf. J. Chevalier and A. Gheerbrant, *Dictionnaire des Symboles*, Vol. 2, p. 165.

80. In terms of the various personifications of a man's anima, she would be a Sophia figure. (Cf. page 94)

81. "On the Psychology of the Unconscious," in *Two Essays on Analytical Psychology*, CW 7, par. 32.

82. Brod, op. cit., p. 108.

83. Janouch, op. cit., p. 179.

84. *Letters to Milena*, p. 171.

85. Brod, op. cit., p. 116.

86. *Letters to Milena*, p. 171.

87. Von Franz, *C.G. Jung, His Myth in Our Time*, pp. 135-136.

88. *Symbols of Transformation*, CW 5, par. 245.

89. *Psychology and Alchemy*, CW 12, pars. 397-398.

90. *Mysterium Coniunctionis*, CW 14, pars. 738ff. The first stage of the *coniunctio* is analogous psychologically to the process of coming to terms with the shadow. The alchemist Gerhard Dorn called this "free-

ing the soul from the fetters of the body," which Jung interprets as "a withdrawal of the naive projections by which we have moulded both the reality around us and the image of our own character." (Ibid., par. 738)

91. Ibid., par. 778.

92. *Aion*, CW 9, II, par. 357.

93. *Psychology and Alchemy*, CW 12, par. 563.

94. "The Psychology of the Transference," in *The Practice of Psychotherapy*, CW 16, par. 489.

95. *The Visions Seminars*, pp. 337-338.

96. "He," in *The Great Wall of China*, p. 140.

97. Ibid., p. 149.

98. Brod, op. cit., pp. 147-148.

99. Ibid., p. 98.

100. "He," in *The Great Wall of China*, p. 134.

101. John Hayward (ed.), *The Penguin Book of Modern Verse*, p. 168.

102. "He," in *The Great Wall of China*, p. 135.

103. "Psychology and Religion," in *Psychology and Religion*, CW 11, pars. 90, 109.

104. *Letter to His Father*, p. 113.

105. Ibid., p. 115.

106. Ibid., p. 113.

107. Richard Wilhelm (transl.), op. cit., p. 232.

108. Von Franz, *The Problem of the Puer Aeternus*, p. VI/13.

109. *The Visions Seminars*, p. 504.

110. Janouch, op. cit., p. 178.

111. "Tractatus aureus," *Ars chemica*, p. 12. (Quoted by Jung in *Psychology and Alchemy*, CW 12, par. 192n)

112. Von Franz, *The Problem of the Puer Aeternus*, p. VIII/16.

113. *Dream Analysis*, Vol. I, pp. 209-210.

114. Cf. Jung, *Symbols of Transformation*, CW 5, pars. 308ff.

115. Ibid., par. 306.

116. *The Visions Seminars*, p. 79.

117. Von Franz, *The Problem of the Puer Aeternus*, p. I/2.

118. "The Provisional Life," in *Analytical Psychology and the English Mind*, p. 75.

119. Ibid.

120. Von Franz and James Hillman, *Lectures on Jung's Typology*, p. 33.

121. H.K. Fierz, "The Clinical Significance of Introversion and Extraversion," in *Current Trends in Analytical Psychology*, p. 91.

122. R.B. Onians, *The Origins of European Thought*, pp. 13-14, 23.

123. Janouch, op. cit., p. 23.

124. *The Visions Seminars*, p. 95.

125. Baynes, op. cit., p. 69 (my italics).

126. *Letter to His Father*, p. 73.

127. Von Franz, *The Problem of the Puer Aeternus*, p. VIII/9.

128. "A Psychological Approach to the Dogma of the Trinity," in *Psychology and Religion*, CW 11, par. 276.

129. Janouch, op. cit., p. 23.

130. "Reflections," in *The Great Wall of China*, pp. 143-144.

131. "Psychological Aspects of the Mother Archetype," in *The Archetypes and the Collective Unconscious*, CW 9,I, par. 164.

132. Ibid.

133. Ibid., par. 165.

134. Calvin S. Hall and Richard E. Lind, *Dreams, Life, and Literature, A Study of Franz Kafka*, p. 82.

135. Cf. especially Brod, op. cit., pp. 52ff, 63ff, 100ff.

136. H.E. Jacob, "Truth for Truth's Sake," in *The Kafka Problem*, p. 54.

137. Brod, op. cit., p. 170.

138. Ibid., p. 97.

139. Ibid., p. 95.

140. *Aion*, CW 9, II, par. 22.

141. "Psychological Factors Determining Human Behaviour," in *The Structure and Dynamics of the Psyche*, CW 8, par. 245.

142. "Reflections," in *The Great Wall of China*, p. 145.

143. Ibid., p. 142.

144. "The Psychology of the Transference," in *The Practice of Psychotherapy*, CW 16, par. 400.

145. Henry Miller, *The Wisdom of the Heart*, p. 24.

146. "Archetypes of the Collective Unconscious," in *The Archetypes and the Collective Unconscious*, CW 9,I, par. 66.

147. Cf. von Franz, "The Process of Individuation," in *Man and His Symbols*, pp. 185-186.

148. "The Philosophical Tree," in *Alchemical Studies,* CW 13, par. 454.

149. Ibid., par. 455.

150. *Symbols of Transformation,* CW 5, par. 569.

151. Cf. A.R. Pope, *The Eros Aspect of the Eye.*

152. Onians, op. cit., pp. 233, 235-236.

153. Jung, "Definitions," in *Psychological Types,* CW 6, par. 801.

154. *Aion,* CW 9,II, par. 126.

155. Harry Slochower, *A Kafka Miscellany,* p. 110.

156. Brod, op. cit., p. 186.

157. Janouch, op. cit., pp. 53-54.

158. "The Psychology of the Child Archetype," in *The Archetypes and the Collective Unconscious,* CW 9,I, par. 287.

159. Ibid., par. 285.

160. Ibid., par. 288.

161. *The Great Wall of China,* p. 133.

162. Cf. Emma Jung and Marie-Louise von Franz, *The Grail Legend,* pp. 82-83.

163. Any conflict situation constellates the archetype of the hostile brothers, the paradigm of which (in the Judaic-Christian tradition) is the Cain and Abel myth. (Cf. Jung, "A Psychological Approach to the Dogma of the Trinity," in *Psychology and Religion,* CW 11, pars. 254ff) The resolution (or not) of this conflict through "the feminine" is the subject of E. Fraser Boa, *The Two Brothers,* "A Psychological Exploration of the Cain and Abel Symbolism with Particular Reference to *East of Eden* by John Steinbeck." (Cf. especially "The Positive Feminine," pp. 65ff)

164. She was working in a holiday camp of the Berlin Jewish People's Home. (Cf. Brod, op. cit., p. 196)

165. Cf. Ad de Vries, *Dictionary of Symbols and Imagery,* pp. 188-190.

166. Brod, op. cit., p. 197.

167. Ibid.

168. Ibid., pp. 196-213.

169. "He," in *The Great Wall of China,* p. 134.

170. "Psychology and Religion," in *Psychology and Religion,* CW 11, par. 9.

171. "A Psychological Approach to the Dogma of the Trinity," ibid., par. 260.

172. Thus Erich Heller points out that in Kafka "we have before us the modern mind . . . . he knows two things at once, and both with equal assurance: that there *is* no God, and that there *must* be God." (*The Disinherited Mind*, p. 181)
173. "The Tavistock Lectures," in *The Symbolic Life*, CW 18, pars. 388-389.
174. Cf. Onians, op. cit., p. 233; also de Vries, op. cit., p. 470.
175. "A Psychological Approach to the Dogma of the Trinity," in *Psychology and Religion*, CW 11, par. 276.
176. *Letter to His Father*, p. 11.
177. Brod, op. cit., p. 78.
178. "On Psychic Energy," in *The Structure and Dynamics of the Psyche*, CW 8, par. 66.
179. Ibid., par. 69.
180. *Symbols of Transformation*, CW 5, par. 438.
181. Peter T. Furst, "The Shamanic Universe," in *Stones, Bones, and Skin: Ritual and Shamanic Art*, p. 43.
182. De Vries, op. cit., pp. 199-200.
183. Cf. Anne Maguire, *The Organ of the Skin as the Somatic Vehicle of Psychic Expression*.

## Bibliography

Baynes, H.G. *Analytical Psychology and the English Mind*, Methuen, London, 1950.

Boa, E. Fraser. *The Two Brothers*, Diploma Thesis, C.G. Jung Institute, Zürich, 1977.

Brod, Max. *Franz Kafka, A Biography*, Schocken Books, New York, 1963.

Chevalier, J., and A. Gheerbrant. *Dictionnaire des Symboles*, 4 vols., Seghers, Paris, 1969.

Dale-Green, Patricia. *Dog*, Rupert Hart-Davis, London, 1966.

De Vries, Ad. *Dictionary of Symbols and Imagery*, Elsevier, Amsterdam, 1974.

Fierz, H.K. "The Clinical Significance of Introversion and Extraversion," in *Current Trends in Analytical Psychology* (Proceedings of the First International Congress for Analytical Psychology, 1958), G. Adler (ed.), Tavistock Press, London, 1961.

Flores, Angel (ed.). *The Kafka Problem*, New Directions, New York, 1946.

Fraiberg, Selma. "Kafka and the Dream," in Wm. Philips (ed.), *Art and Psychoanalysis*, World Publishing Co., Cleveland, 1963.

Furst, Peter T. "The Shamanic Universe," in *Stones, Bones and Skin: Ritual and Shamanic Art*, Arts Canada (30th Anniversary Issue), Toronto, 1973.

Greenberg, Martin. *The Terror of Art*, Basic Books, New York, 1968.

Hall, Calvin S., and Richard E. Lind. *Dreams, Life, and Literature, A Study of Franz Kafka*, University of N.C. Press, Chapel Hill, 1970.

Hayward, John (ed.). *The Penguin Book of Modern Verse*, Penguin Books, London, 1956.

Heller, Erich. *The Disinherited Mind*, Pelican Books, London, 1961.

Jacob, H.E. "Truth for Truth's Sake," in Angel Flores (ed.), *The Kafka Problem*, New Directions, New York, 1946.

Janouch, Gustav. *Conversations with Kafka*, transl. Goronwy Rees, Andre Deutsch, London, 1971.

Jung, C.G. *The Collected Works* (Bollingen Series XX), 20 vols., transl. R.F.C. Hull, ed. H. Read, M. Fordham, G. Adler, Wm. McGuire, Princeton U.P., Princeton, 1953-1979.

_____. *Dream Analysis* (Notes of the Seminars, 1928-1930), 2 vols., Psychological Club, Zürich, 1972.

_____. *Letters* (Bollingen Series XCV), 2 vols., ed. G. Adler, Princeton U. P., Princeton, 1973-1975.

_____. *The Visions Seminars* (Notes of the Seminars, 1930-1934), Spring Publications, Zürich, 1976.

Jung, Emma, and Marie-Louise von Franz. *The Grail Legend*, G.P. Putnam's Sons, New York, 1970.

Kafka, Franz. *The Diaries of Franz Kafka*, 1910-1913 (transl. Joseph Kresh) and 1914-1923 (transl. Martin Greenberg), ed. Max Brod, Secker & Warburg, London, 1948-1949.

_____. *The Great Wall of China and Other Pieces*, transl. Willa and Edwin Muir, Secker & Warburg, London, 1946.

_____. *Letter to His Father*, transl. Ernst Kaiser and Eithne Wilkins, Schocken Books, New York, 1966.

_____ *Letters to Milena*, transl. Tania and James Stern, Schocken Books, New York, 1962.

_____. *The Penal Colony* (Stories and Short Pieces), transl. Willa and Edwin Muir, Schocken Books, New York, 1961.

————. *Wedding Preparations in the Country and Other Posthumous Writings*, Secker & Warburg, London, 1954.

Kaufmann, Walter (ed.). *Nietzsche*, Viking Portable, New York, 1954.

Maguire, Anne. *The Organ of the Skin as the Somatic Vehicle of Psychic Expression*, Diploma Thesis, C.G. Jung Institute, Zürich, 1975.

Mann, Thomas. *Tonio Kröger*, Penguin Books, London, 1955.

Miller, Henry. *The Wisdom of the Heart*, New Directions, New York, 1950.

Onians, R.B. *The Origins of European Thought* (Reprint of the 1951 edition), Arno Press, New York, 1973.

Phillips, Wm. (ed.). *Art and Psychoanalysis*, Meridian Books, World Publishing Co., Cleveland, 1963.

Pope, A.R. *The Eros Aspect of the Eye*, C.G. Jung Institute, Zürich, 1968.

Slochower, Harry. *A Kafka Miscellany*, Twice A Year Press, New York, 1940.

Von Franz, Marie-Louise. *C.G. Jung, His Myth in Our Time*, transl. Wm. H. Kennedy, Hodder & Stoughton, London, 1975.

————. *Individuation in Fairytales*, Spring Publications, Zürich, 1971.

————, and James Hillman. *Lectures on Jung's Typology*, Spring Publications, Zürich, 1971.

————. *The Problem of the Puer Aeternus*, Spring Publications, Zürich, 1970.

————. *A Psychological Interpretation of the Golden Ass of Apuleius*, Spring Publications, Zürich, 1970.

————. "The Process of Individuation," in *Man and His Symbols*, ed. C.G. Jung, Aldus Books, London, 1964.

————, and Emma Jung. *The Grail Legend*, G.P. Putnam's Sons, New York, 1970.

Wilhelm, Richard (transl.). *The I Ching or Book of Changes*, Routledge & Kegan Paul, London, 1968.

# Index